beauty
secrets

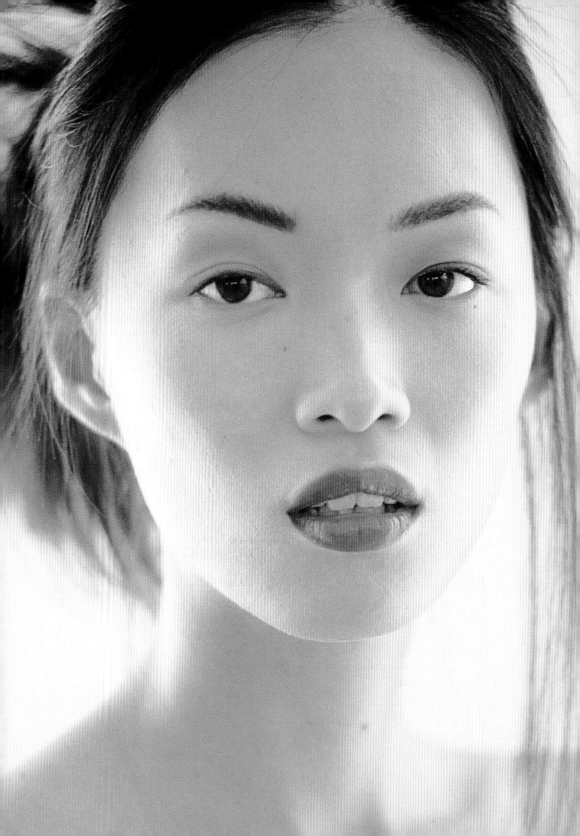

Wendy Lewis

beauty secrets

an insider's guide to the latest skin, hair and body treatments

Quadrille

Editorial Director: **Jane O'Shea**

Creative Director: **Mary Evans**

Designer: **Sue Storey**

Project Editor: **Lisa Pendreigh**

Editor: **Katy Ginn**

Editorial Assistant: **Jaine Keskeys**

Picture Research: **Nadine Bazar**

Illustrations: **Sue Storey**

Production Director: **Vincent Smith**

Production: **Beverley Richardson**

This edition first published in 2004 by
Quadrille Publishing Limited
Alhambra House
27–31 Charing Cross Road
London WC2H 0LS

Before following any advice or practice suggested in this book, it is recommended that
you consult your doctor as to its suitability, especially if you suffer from any health problems
or special conditions. The publishers, the author and the photographers cannot accept
responsibility for any injuries or damage incurred as a result of following the exercises in
this book or of using any of the therapeutic methods described or mentioned here.

Cataloguing-in-Publication Data: a catalogue record for this book is available from the British Library.

ISBN 1 84400 093 1

Printed in China

Contents

Beauty Secrets *is the result of my endeavours to distil the two decades I have spent researching the field in the UK, America and abroad, and the extensive knowledge I have accumulated from recognised experts about the skin, hair and body. I counsel hundreds of women (and men too) who are confused and misinformed about cosmetic enhancements. They are eager to take the plunge, but they just don't have the knowledge to do so safely. My mission is to arm you with vital information and resources previously available only from the very top Dermatologists and Cosmetic Surgeons around the world. I have interviewed countless doctors on both sides of the pond to get the scoop without the hype on the very best treatments, procedures and products on the market.*

There have been three major advances in the arena of beauty and anti-ageing treatments in recent years – botulinum toxin, liposuction and lasers, which have become mainstream because they are effective at forestalling more invasive surgical intervention. Let's face it, we all want to erase our flaws and imperfections without surgery if we can. This book reveals the key non-surgical options for you, the advantages and disadvantages, and what results you can expect and what they simply cannot do for you. In addition to smart prevention and maintenance tips, in Beauty Secrets, I share with you the most state-of-the-art solutions science has to offer, so you know what works and what is just a waste of your precious time and money.

In compiling Beauty Secrets, I listened to my private clients from around the world and noted their chief concerns. Women have the same complaints and issues no matter where they call home. You will find new tips about common beauty and health topics throughout the book including skin cancer, hyperpigmentation, thread veins, post pregnancy shape up, stretch marks and hair removal.

I am a big believer that any skin can be improved, but it takes solid information and consistent use of the right formulas and lifestyle changes. Don't despair. It won't happen overnight, but you can see marked improvements in disfiguring spots, acne scars, dreaded lines and wrinkles, brown spots, brittle hair and even the appearance of cellulite. With continuous practice, your complexion can be clear and smooth and look more uniform in colour and texture. You can like the way you look. I want to empower you to look as good as possible and even better than your chronological age.

There is no miracle product or treatment out there yet, but we're getting closer every day. Technology is continually developing to give us the tools we need to look and feel beautiful forever. It's just a matter of time.

Stay gorgeous!

Wendy Lewis

wlbeauty@aol.com

www.wlbeauty.com

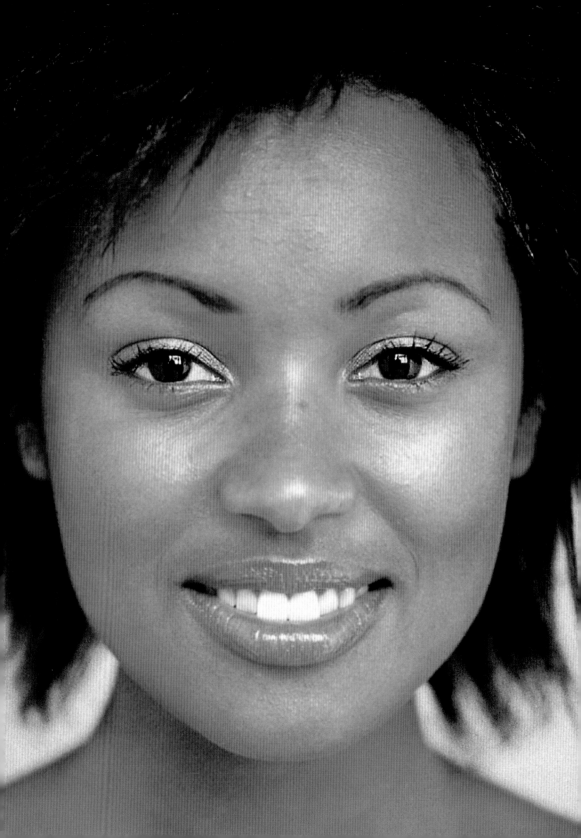

COMPLEXION PERFECTION

Hormonal and other internal upheavals have a way of leaving their mark on your skin in the form of spots, skin eruptions and other lumps and bumps. Acne is the most common skin disease, but only 7 per cent of the 70 million sufferers ever see a dermatologist for help. Acne is a build-up of dried oil and dead skin cells in the hair follicles under the skin. Hormones, particularly male hormones called androgens, stimulate the hormone-sensitive sebaceous glands, which produce sebum. As with many other skin conditions, genetics plays a part. All of these factors work together to start the vicious acne cycle.

If spots are a major problem in your life, join the club. Getting the odd spot is to be expected: we all have oil glands and sometimes they get clogged. The good news is that help is at hand. Whether you have an occasional flare-up or chronic acne that makes you want to hide, there are many effective treatment options. There's still no cure, with or without a prescription. The secret to controlling it is PREVENTION. Most acne therapies require ongoing treatment to keep your skin clear. Even after blemishes disappear, using an effective acne treatment will keep new ones from forming. The first step is determining the type and cause of your acne, then tailoring a skin-care protocol that targets it.

demystifying spots

demystifying spots

Although spots come in a variety of forms, all pimples start out the same – as a plugged-up follicle. They actually begin 2-3 weeks before the blemishes show up on your face.

Blackheads are formed when dead skin cells and sebum are packed inside a follicle where the walls have broken. If the plug enlarges and pops out of the duct, it's a blackhead.

Whiteheads are formed on or under the skin, showing up as a skin-coloured or inflamed bump. The opening of the plugged sebaceous follicle is closed or very narrow, instead of open. With inflammatory acne, whiteheads become infected with bacteria, causing them to swell.

Papules are red, raised bumps or inflamed lesions that occur when oily materials inside the follicle rupture into the skin. They show up as small, solid lesions, slightly elevated above the surface of the skin.

Pustules are dome-shaped lesions similar to papules but inflamed with pus. Pustules formed over sebaceous follicles usually have a hair in the centre. Pustules that heal without turning into a cystic form don't usually scar.

Cysts are a severe form of inflammatory acne – closed, hard sacs that can be large and painful. A cyst extends into the deeper layers of the skin where they can destroy tissue structures and cause scarring.

spotting causes

spotting causes

Acne is often linked to genetics and stress. Adding hormones to the mix can really defeat your skin. Getting to the root of the problem can be a challenge.

Hormones – specifically androgens produced by the ovaries and adrenal glands in women – trigger most acne attacks. Androgens cause sebaceous glands to enlarge; when they get over-stimulated, acne flares up. Acne can crop up any time hormones are in flux, during puberty, pregnancy or menopause. Odd pimples showing up every month is not necessarily acne.

Oil production increases as sebaceous glands are stimulated by androgens; oil accumulates in the follicle and travelling up hair shafts to the skin's surface. As it travels, it mixes with bacteria and dead skin cells shed from the lining of the follicle. The greater the oil production, the greater the likelihood that the hair follicle will become clogged and result in spots.

Follicle changes occur as androgen levels increase and sebaceous glands enlarge. Normally, dead cells inside the follicle are expelled onto the surface. During hormonal flux, these cells are shed more rapidly and stick together. When mixed with sebum, they clog the follicle and form a plug.

Bacteria breeds wildly in clogged sebaceous glands and follicles. *Propionibacterium acnes (P. acnes)* multiply rapidly and chemicals produced by the bacteria can cause inflammation in the follicle and surrounding skin.

raging hormones

Once you've survived the awkward teenage years – braces, cramming for tests, bad school photos – you would expect to have left pimples and problem skin behind.

If you've been dealing with breakouts since your teens, you've probably heard things like 'Don't worry, lots of kids your age go through this' or 'You'll grow out of it.' While many teens suffering from spots eventually get clear, sometimes spot prone skin remains longer or may not even start until adulthood. Perhaps you sailed through your teens with perfect skin, only to start breaking out in your 20s, 30s or 40s.

REALITY CHECK: Oily skin tends to develop lines and wrinkles at a slower rate, so your oily skin may actually be keeping your skin looking younger for longer.

Many cases of acne accompany the hormonal changes of pregnancy, irregularities in the menstrual cycle or ovarian cysts, which may increase androgen productivity. Women typically suffer from adult onset or worsening acne more often than men, and they may have the problem for many years. Stress almost always plays a role because it stimulates the gland that produces androgens. When you feel stressed, your hormone levels fluctuate, which can cause increased oil production in the skin. Most of us notice an extra blemish or two before a major event in our lives, which is, of course, the worst possible timing. Don't panic. Get serious about how to control it.

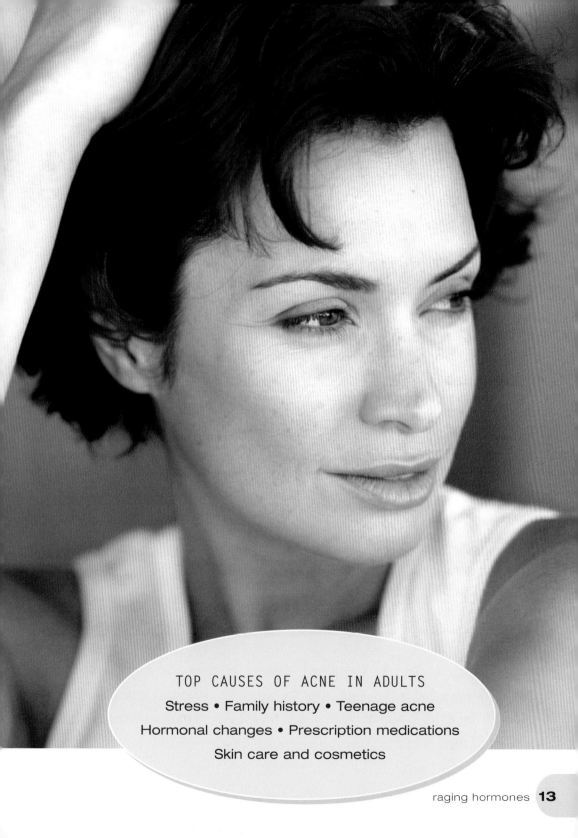

TOP CAUSES OF ACNE IN ADULTS

Stress • Family history • Teenage acne
Hormonal changes • Prescription medications
Skin care and cosmetics

spot cycle

Hormonal medications and endocrine disorders are cited as causes of acne flare-ups in grown women. Many women experience monthy outbreaks caused by the release of progesterone after ovulation.

Even slight hormonal fluctuations can increase the number of new pimples, blackheads and whiteheads, as well as the oiliness of the forehead and cheeks. This is most common at about 5 days before the beginning of the cycle and continues for 7–10 days. Learn to adjust your skin care regime to account for these monthly fluctuations.

Some women are genetically prone to drastic hormone swings, have higher levels of androgens and oil glands that are more sensitive to hormones. Your doctor may recommend taking an oral contraceptive to change the balance between androgenic and female hormones to help control acne breakouts. Oral contraceptives change your hormone levels, and can cause breakouts both when started and stopped. Some birth control pills are specially formulated to control acne. Ortho Tri-Cyclen has a combination of ethinyl oestradiol, a synthetic oestrogen, and norgestimate, a progestin. Other formulations with a low amount of androgen can be used to treat acne. They reduce sebum production significantly, leading to beneficial effects in skin and hair. For example, Dianette contains a small dose of Cyproterone Acetate combined with the female type hormone ethinyloestradiol (an oestrogen). Cyproterone Acetate also inhibits the production of oestrogen. The addition of ethinyloestradiol compensates for the lack of oestrogen and the menopausal-type symptoms that would otherwise result. It is usually taken for 12-36 months.

Yasmin is a new birth control pill with dual-property progestin, drospirenone, which is similar to Spironolactone, an anti-androgenm commonly used to treat acne. The pill may not be effective at all, or only for a certain period of time. For some lucky women, it can be the answer to their acne woes. Improvement doesn't necessarily mean an end to complexion worries. It can be combined with standard acne treatments like retinoids and antibiotics for maximum effectiveness. If bacteria enter into the picture and inflammation and redness become evident, more aggressive treatments such as oral antibiotics may be necessary. The pill can also have side effects including weight gain, blood clots, heart attack, stroke, hypertension and diabetes. These risks are higher in women who smoke and increase with age.

Your gynaecologist might suggest blood tests or an ultrasound to pinpoint any underlying hormonal imbalances that could be a contributing factor to your acne. Irregular periods, excess facial hair, weight gain, infertility, oily skin and acne can each be a sign of polycystic ovary syndrome (PCOS). Excess production of androgenic hormones may be causing these effects.

BEAUTY BYTES:

For information on PCOS, go to

www.verity-pcos.org.uk

teen troubles

When your skin is spotty and shiny, you feel like you just want to hide. The best bet for teens is to take the fast track to oil control and get with the programme.

- Got blackheads? Get a vitamin A derivative, like retinoic acid, to get deep into oil plugs and stop clogged pores.

- Don't over-coat your face with acne medications – use only a thin layer to avoid irritation and redness.

- If you can feel hard lumps deep under the skin, see a consultant dermatologist. Don't self-treat.

- Less is more – don't overdo the scrubbing, massaging, or cleansing. Be gentle.

- Don't touch your face more than you absolutely have to. Hands can spread bacteria and cause breakouts.

- Don't get discouraged if a treatment isn't working. Seek advice about switching to something that may be more effective.

- Once you find that magic combination that keeps your acne under control, stick with it.

- Work to keep skin balanced – a healthy ratio of oily to dry. Don't dry your skin out and don't over-moisturise to compensate for dry patches.

pregnant pores

pregnant pores

If you have a history of acne, your skin may either improve or get worse when you are expecting a child. Acne can appear at any stage during pregnancy and may or may not clear up after childbirth.

When you're pregnant, anything goes. Breakouts can show up on the face, chest, back or elsewhere. Random flare-ups can happen at any time, especially in the first trimester and may level off during the second.

Although prenatal acne cannot be prevented, there are steps you can take to minimise breakouts. Keep your skin in good shape before and after becoming pregnant and practise early intervention. Keep it simple – during pregnancy, skin reactivity changes a lot and your skin may be sensitive to certain ingredients. Some glycolic acid products are considered safe for use by pregnant women, but most common acne treatments are a no go.

Whatever is done to the mother may affect the foetus. Medications like antibiotics, vitamin A derivatives and benzoyl peroxide should not be used by pregnant women or resumed until the baby is weaned. Salicylic acid (Beta hydroxy acid) is not generally recommended, as it is absorbed through the skin and can interfere with blood clotting. These drugs fall under the US FDA 'Pregnancy Category C', meaning that animal studies have not been conducted and it is unknown whether they can harm the foetus or if the drug is excreted in human milk. The final decision should always be left to your obstetrician or paediatrician.

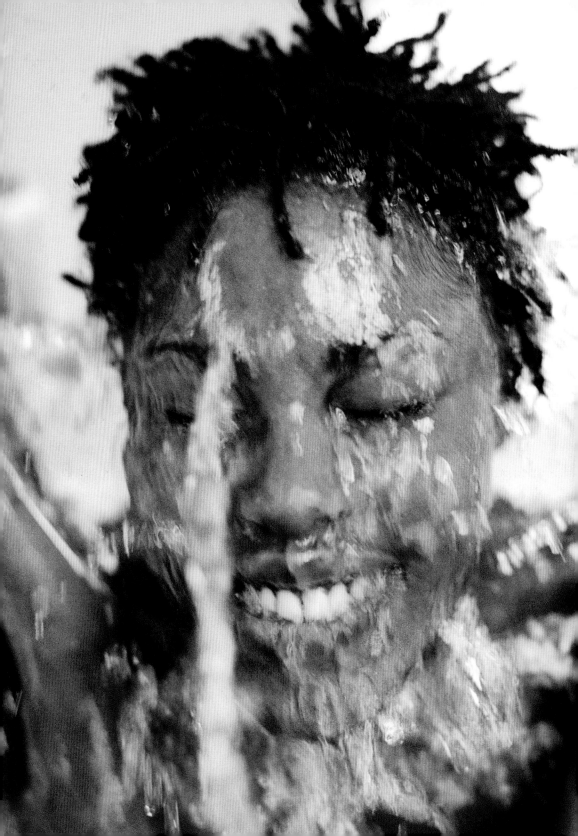

OIL PATROL

OIL PATROL

Forget what you've been hearing for ages. The secret to reducing your shine lies more in what you put on your skin than what you put into your body. Contrary to popular myth, controlling oil glands is not food related, so following a strictly no-grease diet won't clear your skin. While gorging on chips, chocolate and other greasy foods may not cause acne, it won't do wonders for the way your clothes fit. Drinking lots of water won't really help acne either, even though it is good for you in other ways.

As with all things skin related, do what works for you. Some women swear they break out after consuming chocolate, ketchup, or cola. Avoiding allergenic substances such as dairy, caffeine and alcohol is sometimes recommended. Excessive iodine, found in fast foods, milk and shellfish, has been cited as an acne trigger. It may be prudent to avoid any foods that seem to aggravate spots, as a precaution. No one knows your skin as well as you do.

The same applies to skin-care products. When you hit upon the right formula, stick to it. The trick is to eliminate excess shine without stripping the skin of its natural oils. Choose non-comedogenic cleansers, moisturisers and cosmetics specially formulated for oily skin only. Clear skin is the BEST accessory – it goes with everything!

squeaky clean

squeaky clean

You can't scrub spots away. Cleansing overload can aggravate pimples and slow down the healing process. The key is using just enough of the right products.

Work gently to unclog pores and fight bacteria that causes the micro-infection which turns into acne. It is natural to want to overexfoliate to wage war on every drop of oil in the skin, but this can trigger breakouts, as your oil glands overcompensate. Acne doesn't necessarily mean your face is dirty. If you aren't washing thoroughly enough, dirt can clog pores and cause pimples. If you are constantly stripping away essential oils that your skin can't replace, you may be drying out the surface layer and making your skin less able to hold its own moisture. If your skin is dry, it will produce more oil, which becomes trapped in your pores. It's a vicious cycle.

Don't use soap, which can dry out the skin. Use a pea-sized amount of soap-free, scent-free cleanser and wash your face from under the jaw to the hairline. Thoroughly rinse to get rid of any film from the cleanser. Non-alcohol astringents should be used only on oily areas. If your skin gets shiny or doesn't feel clean without them, try using alpha-hydroxy acid cleansing pads that mildly exfoliate, clear and refresh oily skin. Organic loofahs and sea sponges may harbour bacteria, whereas non-organic textured sponges fo not carry this risk.

TOP TIP:
Always use a fresh washcloth to avoid bacteria that can grow in damp cloths.

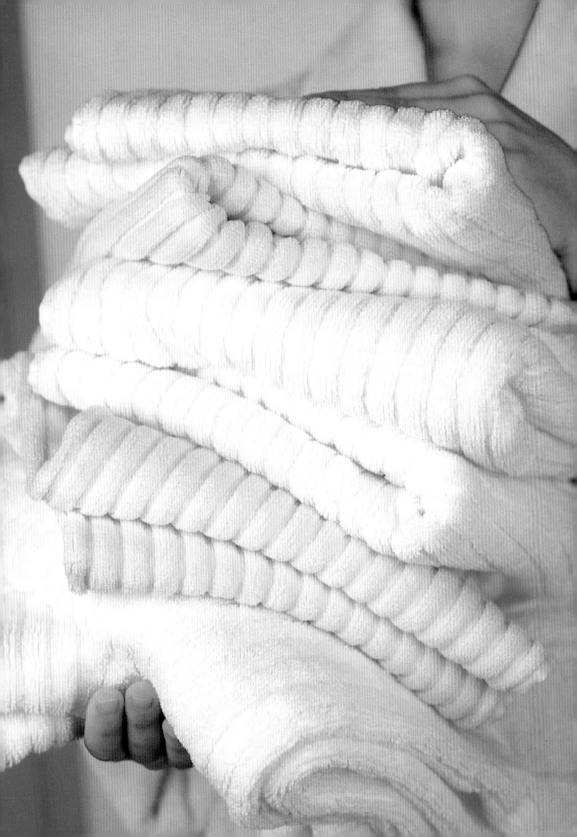

balancing act

Acne and dry skin can co-exist on the same face. Acne treatments can be very drying, especially if you have sensitive skin or eczema to start with. The key is to strike a balance.

Dry skin indicates that it is lacking oil; dehydrated skin means a lack of water. Oily skin can be dehydrated even though it has plenty of oil. If you attempt to strip skin of all its oil content, you may end up with skin that is even oilier. Look for words like 'mild', 'nonirritating' and 'nondrying'. Be careful with cleansers that contain medications like salicylic acid. Cleanse first and then apply your medication so you don't layer up, which can be too irritating. If you get red and flaky, skip a day or two before using your medication again, so your skin can heal.

The 'T-zone' runs from the forehead down the nose to the chin, where oil glands are most plentiful. Some surface grease on the skin is normal – it lubricates the skin's outer layer, keeping it protected. Most people see the bulk of it on the forehead and nose, the most common locations for acne. Humidity and high temperatures can also wreak havoc on your T-zone. If you're active and enjoy sports, perspiration may add to your shine. Also, avoid standing near foods that are being cooked in oil – flipping burgers and frying chips are a culprit for teenage acne.

To control T-zone breakouts, apply salicylic acid or benzoyl peroxide formulas or both in small amounts to affected areas. Be careful of the chin area, which tends to get especially dry. A matt absorbent powder will also help to soak up excess oil.

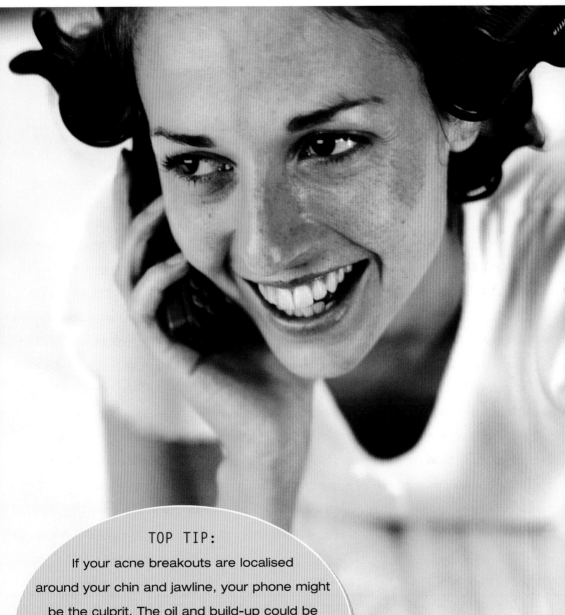

TOP TIP:

If your acne breakouts are localised
around your chin and jawline, your phone might
be the culprit. The oil and build-up could be
irritating your skin. Cleanse the mouthpiece and
receiver every morning with hydrogen peroxide or
alcohol. Don't let the phone rest between your
chin and shoulder and keep it away
from your skin.

tackling outbreaks

Your first course of action is to treat breakouts on your own.
Start by reviewing the products you are currently using.
Your skin-care regime may actually be the culprit.

Every acne sufferer has encountered over-the-counter products that only work for a short while. Blotting out the oil, soaking it up and keeping skin shine-free can be a full-time job.

Many moisturisers, creams and other skin-care and cosmetic products contain fats, oils and waxes that can clog pores and make problem skin worse. Declare a moratorium on any product that feels creamy, heavy or isn't oil-free.

Women who are nearing forty may feel inclined to focus on moisturisation and as a result, overload their skin with pore-clogging ingredients such as lanolin, cocoa butter, sesame oil, and avocado oil. Gels or lighter lotions are better suited to oily skin.

Pore size is genetically determined. Skin type is determined by the degree of oiliness or dryness. Generally, skin type correlates with pore size. The thicker and oilier your skin, the larger and more noticeable your pores will be.

Nothing has been proven to permanently shrink pores. Keeping pores clean and unplugged can make them look smaller. Pore strips may help, but they really can't go deep enough to extract the gunk that's buried. You can prevent the keratinised plug from forming with good exfoliation. Masks that contain kaolin, calamine or clay can absorb excess oil, calm the skin and keep pores toned. Shine also draws attention to pore size.

Exfoliation is vital when it comes to caring for oily, spot-prone skin. Figure out if your skin thickness is thin, medium or thick by judging its strength, resiliency, and general condition. Healthy skin is smooth, firm, tight, even, and has good tolerance levels. If your skin is fragile, you need to increase skin thickness by stimulating new collagen, which is what Retin-A does. Thick skin needs to get sloughed to keep its barrier function intact. Look for active concentrations of alpha hydroxy or glycolic and lactic acid, and beta hydroxy (BHA), or salicylic acid, to produce a superficial glow and keep pores unclogged. Higher concentrations will clear skin faster, but start with mild formulas and work your way up.

You may also need to switch some of your cosmetics to oil-free formulas. Lip products that contain moisturisers may cause small open and closed comedos to form. Hairstyling products that come into contact with the hairline can cause breakouts or stinging. Hair dyes that contain coal tar have been cited as potential acne triggers. Other lesser known irritants include fabric softeners, perfume and hair spray. Choose formulas that are non-acnegenic (won't cause acne, pustules, or papules) and noncomedogenic (won't cause comedos, like blackheads or whiteheads). Some products that are labelled non-comedogenic may even cause acne.

> **TOP TIP:**
> An oil-free product can become oil based when it comes into contact with the natural oils in your skin and environmental debris.

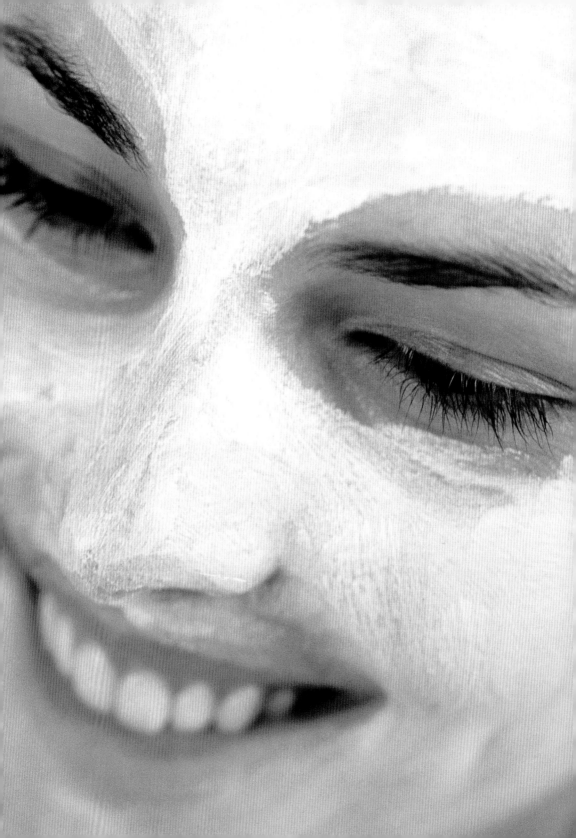

dos and don'ts for perfect skin

- **DO** wash skin with a mild, detergent-free cleanser that doesn't leave a residue, twice daily.

- **DO** use a clay-based mask treatment once a week to eliminate excess oiliness.

- **DO** treat your skin to a series of superficial peels or microdermabrasion treatments to purge pores.

- **DO** avoid rough scrubbing and massage, which can stimulate oil glands.

- **DON'T** pick or squeeze pimples, which can spread infection, delay healing, and cause long-term scarring.

- **DO** rinse with cold water after cleansing and use an alcohol-free toner, especially in humid weather.

- **DO** use a fresh washcloth daily to avoid bacteria that can grow in damp cloths.

- **DO** shampoo hair daily and avoid heavy conditioners, and don't let your hair hang over your face.

- **DON'T** give up too soon. Give therapies at least six weeks to kick in.

- **DO** wash your face after exercising to remove any sweat and dirt.

- **DO** stop touching your face to avoid spreading the bacteria that cause acne.

- **DO** treat blackheads when they first appear to avoid any bigger problems later.

buffed up

If you suffer from acne, choose your skin specialist wisely. Not all therapists are trained in the accurate assessment of problem skin and its special needs.

All acne treatments should be given under sanitary conditions. Mild steam cleansing together with an exfoliation treatment to remove dead topical cells, extractions and a soothing, healing mask is the best course. Facial scrubs that buff away excess oil, dirt and dead skin can also give skin a big boost. However, rubbing and massaging can cause irritation and intense facial massage, rich European-style facial creams and overhandling of delicate pores can aggravate acne and cause eruptions. If your skin looks like it went through a war after a facial treatment, your technician may be too heavy-handed and aggressive.

Milia are deep little white bumps that form like tiny cysts. Exfoliation can help get rid of them by unroofing the skin cells that are trapped and sloughing them away. Whiteheads are closed comedos and should only be extracted in the hands of an expert. A consultant dermatologist may use a sterile needle to prick the tip of the pimple – do not try this at home. When you squeeze spots yourself, you risk making the situation worse. Try applying a salicylic gel or cream to help unplug the pore instead. Holding ice to the area whenever you feel the urge to touch it can help. When acne is treated effectively, squeezing is not neccessary. Treatment interferes with the way acne develops, so spots will clear up on their own.

DIY acne facial

- **Cleansing:** Apply a cleanser with the fingertips and work into the skin. Remove completely with a face cloth.

- **Steaming:** Apply a warm cloth to the face to soften the skin and relax pores.

- **Extraction:** With a tissue around your two fingers, gently squeeze the pore. If the oil plug isn't released, abort the mission. Gently exfoliate with a mild scrub with micro beads.

- **Astringent:** Wipe the skin clean with a mild alcohol-free toner to remove any residue.

- **Mask:** Apply a clay- or mud-based purifying mask. Leave on for ten minutes. Alternatively, use an at-home peel.

- **Spray:** Wipe off the mask with a warm face cloth and follow with a cooling mist to close pores.

Maintenance is important to keep skin clear. A combination of at-home and professional treatments works best.

TOP TIP:
Instead of frequent salon facials that can activate oil glands, switch to microdermabrasion (see page 56).

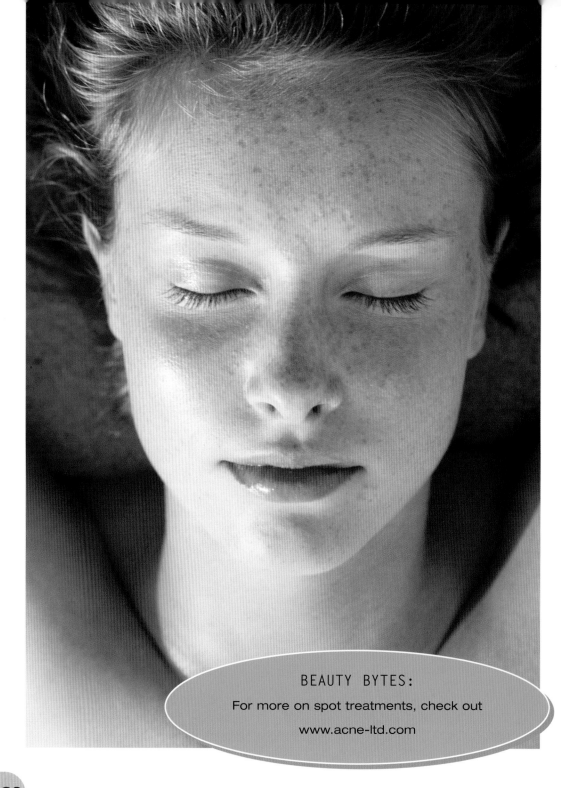

BEAUTY BYTES:

For more on spot treatments, check out

www.acne-ltd.com

sun spots

sun spots

As many as one third of acne sufferers report that summer is the worst time of year for spots. Some women still believe that sunning and sun beds improve their skin.

Warmer weather and humidity can bring on breakouts. Sun creams and lotions can clog pores that are open wide from the heat, so they absorb them more readily. Catching rays will not clear up acne. Small amounts of sun exposure may initially make it better, but continuous sunning can increase plugging of the pores that produce blackheads, whiteheads and small spots.

A tan can temporarily dry up some of the oil, but the drying factor could actually encourage the skin to produce more oil. Prolonged exposure to the sun can worsen the condition. Many acne treatments, especially vitamin A derivatives like RoAccutane and some antibiotics like doxycycline, increase the skin's sensitivity to ultraviolet light, making the risk of sunburn greater. Tanning will darken the lesion, which will make it take much longer to fade away, and post-inflammatory hyperpigmentation.

Use only sun protection products formulated for acne-prone skin and make sure you rinse off all residue from your face and body at the end of the day. An SPF 15 should be used daily for protection for all skin types, even dark complexions. Without it, instead of spots, you'll have more wrinkles. Sun exposure is a lose-lose situation no matter how you look at it.

body beautiful

Spots are not limited to the oily T-zone of the face. They can show up anywhere, any time. Stress and hormones can induce acne lesions on the body, especially the back and chest.

Acne develops where sebaceous glands are most numerous: the face, scalp, neck, chest, back, upper arms, and shoulders. Perspiration and snug clothing are two of the most common causes of body acne, which explains why many physically active women are plagued by it. Tight-fitting fabrics such as spandex trap perspiration against the skin, allowing it to mix with surface oils. The result is a film that clogs pores and causes blemishes ranging from whiteheads to inflamed papules and pustules.

TOP TIP: Avoid creamy hair lotions or wear headbands that can clog pores around the hairline and on the back.

Acne mechanica is a form of acne that is caused by heat, pressure and repetitive frictional rubbing against the skin. It can be the result of wearing tight-fitting synthetic workout clothes, bra straps, and underwear. Place a clean towel down before lying on exercise mats or equipment. Wear clean cotton T-shirts or bras under exercise clothing: Cotton absorbs sweat and reduces friction against the skin. If you sweat through exercise and don't shower immediately afterwards, you are inviting flare-ups. Sweat traps dirt and oil in the pores. High temperatures and humidity act in the same way. At the very least, wash the chest, back, and other areas prone to acne after your workout. Don't go straight to the steam room – shower first to get rid of bacteria.

If you have oily hair, shampoo daily but avoid heavy conditioners or styling products. If you have breakouts on your forehead, having a fringe may be a contributing factor. Style hair so that it is off your face and neck.

Cleansers containing salicylic acid are good for removing surface oils and unclogging pores. Apply an anti-acne medication like a keratolytic solution to eruptions as soon as they appear. High-potency glycolic acid (10–15 per cent) works well on the thicker, tougher skin of the body. Be careful on the chest, which can sometimes be more sensitive. Cleansing pads work well for body areas and may be easier to use.

Therapies for body acne are similar to those for the face, but the former is more resistant to treatment as it is harder to reach. Since you can't see it, you never really know when pores get congested. Have a friend or family member check your back occasionally, or see a professional for regular treatments. You need to treat back acne aggressively, and as skin on the back is tougher, it can take tougher products. 10 per cent benzoyl peroxide wash is often recommended. Continuous treatment with a comedolytic agent such as topical tretinoin may be recommended if back acne persists indefinitely. If inflammatory lesions are present, benzoyl peroxide or topical antibiotics may be added to your regimen. For severe chest and back acne, RoAccutane and steroid injections are indicated.

TOP TIP:

Peroxide can bleach or stain clothing, so if you are using it for back acne, wear an old T-shirt to avoid staining your clothes.

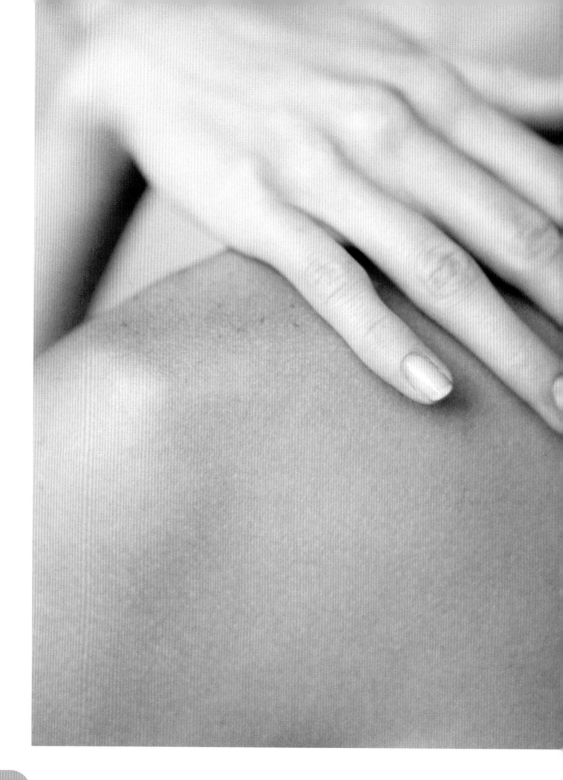

backne regime

backne regime

What could be worse than spots on your back that show up just when you want to wear a skimpy top? If you're prone to back breakouts, ask a friend to check out hard to reach areas that you can't get to on your own.

- **DO** pat dry. Don't wipe or rub vigorously, as this can irritate.

- **DO** wash twice daily with an anti-acne type cleanser.

- **DO** wipe the affected area with a acne treatment pad containing salicylic acid.

- **DO** follow with an alpha hydroxy acid body lotion to help exfoliate skin while preventing it from drying out.

- **DO** use a benzoyl peroxide treatment on individual spots at night or twice a day as needed.

- **DON'T** pick or squeeze spots on the back or chest, where the skin is thicker and more prone to scarring.

- **DON'T** forget to shower as soon as possible after perspiring from sports or activity and wear clean clothes.

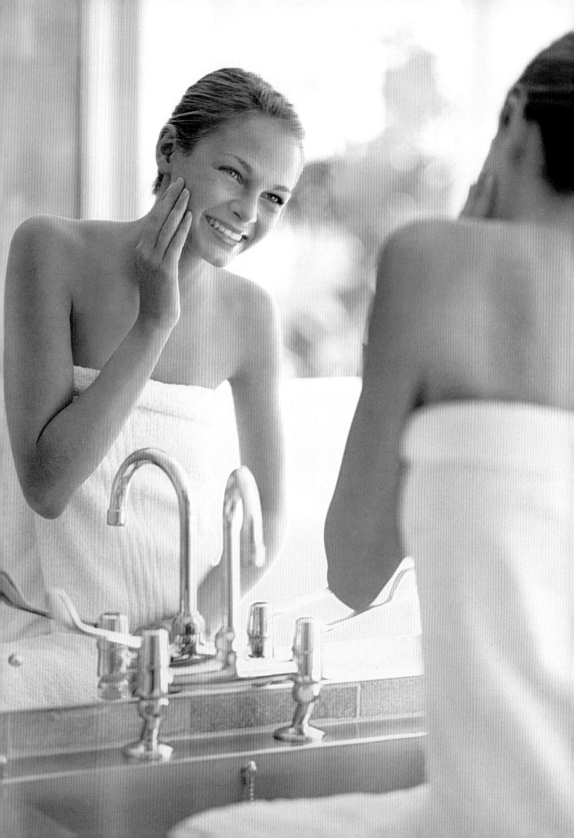

BANISHING BLEMISHES

BANISHING BLEMISHES

No one has to suffer with acne. Help is available in many forms. Effective over-the-counter treatments have taken centre stage and are the most sensible place to start. Finding a treatment best suited to your needs can take a lot of experimentation. Using too much or the wrong type of formula can give your face a shiny look and clog pores.

Treatments for mild to moderate acne reduce the amount of oil produced and the bacteria that cause infection. Anti-bacterials prevent infection spreading. Anti-inflammatories reduce swelling, redness and inflammation. Keratolytics normalise the shedding follicle linings and remove dead cells. Of the nonprescription treatment options available, oil absorbers keep shine to a minimum and drying agents reduce oil plugs and keep pores unclogged.

If you have more sensitive skin and suffer from breakouts, choose your products with caution. 5 per cent tea tree oil applied twice daily is helpful for acne and may be less drying than benzoyl peroxide. Very sensitive skin types may actually develop dermatitis in the form of redness or a rash from tea tree oil, so be careful.

True acne can't be cured completely, but it can be controlled for long periods. It is not uncommon to be in remission for years, and then suffer a flare up at an older age. When your acne is out of control and usual methods no longer work for you, it is time to see your doctor.

drying out

Although there is a huge variety of acne treatments on the market, the majority contain various concentrations of the same key ingredients.

Prescription and over-the-counter benzoyl peroxide treatments work in the same way but prescription formulas often have higher concentrations. It is prescribed most often to make sure patients get the best formulation for their type of acne, either a cream, gel or lotion. Benzoyl peroxide kills bacteria and reduces oil production. Salicylic acid, sulfur and resourcinol help dissolve blackheads and whiteheads. Topical medicines, such as over-the-counter creams and gels are applied directly onto the spotty or spot-prone areas. Most of these help to dry out the excess oil and block the spread of infection. For mild acne, doctors often recommend using an over-the-counter remedy before resorting to more serious treatments that require a prescription. Be patient. It may take a month to see results from over-the-counter products.

Benzoyl peroxide
Concentration 2.5, 5, 10
Kills bacteria, removes shedding cells from follicle

Benzoyl peroxide – destroys the *P. acnes* bacteria by penetrating the follicle and releasing hydrogen peroxide. For more than just a few spots, spread a thin film of cream or ointment over the entire area to prevent the acne from spreading. Benzoyl peroxide's main drawback is that it can cause irritation, dryness, peeling, or redness, and many women stop using it for that reason.

Salicylic acid – found in creams, lotions, and pads. It fights blackheads and whiteheads. Salicylic acid is a beta hydroxy acid that is oil soluble and can therefore penetrate oil-plugged pores. It works by destroying the plug and shedding the cells lining the follicles. You must use salicylic acid treatments continually in order to reap the benefits, as pores clog up again once you stop.

Sulphur – in creams and lotions, sulphur acts as a drying agent by reducing bacteria to help unclog pores and control whiteheads and inflamed pimples.

Sulphur/Resourcinol – can be found in creams and lotions and is usually combined with salicylic acid or benzoyl peroxide to unclog pores.

Glycolic acids – are able to remove excess oils and any surface debris to unclog pores.

sensitivity training

Sensitive skin can mean different things to different people. At one time or another, your skin may be sensitive. It can occur in all skin types, age groups, sexes and seasons.

You may just be born with sensitive skin, which tends to be fair, delicate, and sunburns easily. You may also experience some of these symptoms at various periods in your life due to changes in your emotional and physical wellbeing and lifestyle. Reactive complexions can respond to climate, environmental factors, fatigue, and stress. Heat and sweating, low humidity, cold air, and allergies can also be irritants. Sensitive skin can be prone to blemishes, flakiness, blotchy patches, rashes, chafing, and cracking, and it can feel uncomfortably tight, and burn or sting.

Skin sensitivities can accompany common conditions like atopic dermatitis also called eczema and contact dermatitis, which occur often on the face and scalp. The worst thing you can do to dry, irritated skin is to scratch, which damages the skin, increases inflammation, and may lead to infection. The itch-scratch cycle will surely leave your skin in a weakened state.

Dry skin exacerbates any sensitivities you may have. Skin that is tight and itchy from dryness will be more prone to all kinds of reactions. Generally, the fewer the ingredients, the safer you will be. If your skin is truly sensitive, avoid irritants that can cause inflammation, most notably soaps, detergents, fragrances, colourants, mineral oil and alcohol. Truly sensitive skin can't protect itself in the same way that normal skin can. Stick with formulas that are extra mild with few ingredients. Some women search forever to find a simple regime that will maintain their skin without irritating its sensitive nature.

Use a light textured, oil-free moisturiser and lotions and milks specially developed for reactive skin types. Watch for signs of irritation, and adjust your regime as needed. If you feel a sting, immediately wash off whatever you applied and pat dry. Bathe only with lukewarm water and a detergent-free cleanser or non-alkaline soap. Moisturisers should be applied within a few minutes after getting out of the shower. Using a humidifier may also keep skin protected from extremes. Try spraying a facial mist containing essential oils and hydrating ingredients. Be aware that even 'natural' and 'organic' ingredients can cause irritation in very reactive skin types.

Sensitive skin lacks lipids, which accounts for why it gets easily irritated. Elasticity breaks down and may increase premature aging, but not if you take care of it properly. When the stratum corneum, or outermost layer of cells, that form a barrier to keep moisture in is weakened, the skin's natural defenses become compromised. Irritants like pollution and UV rays can penetrate easier, so sensitive skin needs extra protection to repair the symptoms which can result when the epidermis has been overexposed. Wait until the skin is normalized to get experimental with your skin care.

There seems to be a worldwide explosion of sensitive skin sufferers, perhaps the result of self-treating skin with potent chemicals without the benefit of expert advice. Women often complain about having 'sensitive skin' after one bout of irritation. In response to this growing concern, a fresh crop of non-irritating, fragrance-, chemical- and soap-free formulations has sprouted up that can help nourish reactive, red and irritated skin.

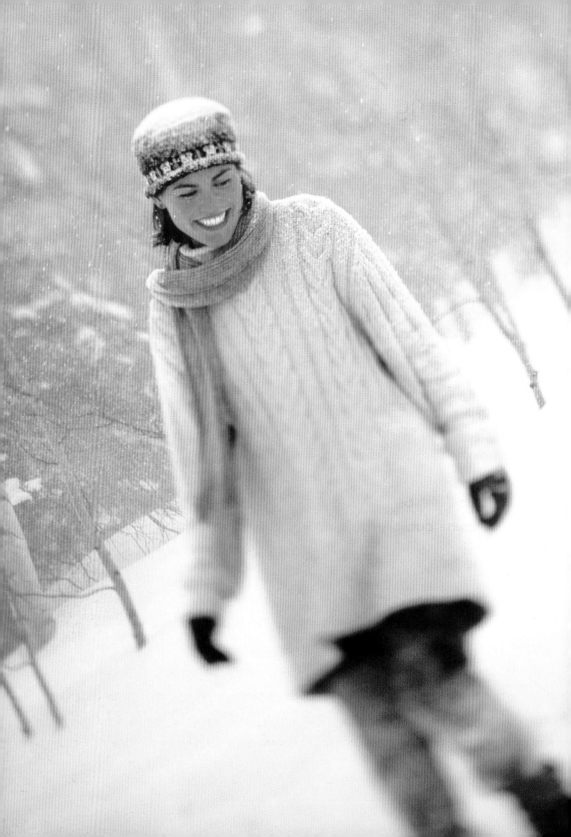

blushing beauty

Your face flushes unexpectedly, the broken blood vessels in your cheeks get red and swollen, you get flare-ups of bumps or pimples, and sometimes a stinging or burning.

These symptoms may last for hours or days and start up without warning. The bad news is that it sounds like rosacea, a chronic skin condition that has no cure. The good news is that rosacea can be treated, and should be. If left untreated, it usually gets worse. Rosacea is generally diagnosed by the stage it is in; first (mild), second (moderate) or third (severe). It starts later in life than acne and affects the cheeks, chin, nose, ears, scalp and forehead. The redness may become ruddier and blood vessels may appear. If left untreated, bumps and spots can develop. In rare cases, the eyes may also look watery, blood shot and irritated.

No cause has been definitively linked with rosacea, which makes it difficult to figure out. It is considered a vascular disorder and can be brought on by menopause, high blood pressure, stress, or fever. Like most skin afflictions, it is more common in women than in men. At least 25 per cent of women in their 30s and 40s have rosacea. Rosacea now ranks as the fifth most common diagnosis made by dermatologists, and it is still considered widely underdiagnosed.

People most prone to rosacea are aged between thirty and sixty, of Irish, English, or Scottish descent, or with northern or eastern European origins, fair skinned, with a family history of rosacea. Having had an adverse reaction to an acne medication or a sty may also be indications.

get the red out

Rosacea is basically a vascular problem, which is why you may appear red and flushed. Thin skin reveals the enlarged veins that lie underneath the surface.

Treatments for rosacea range from topical antibiotics to retinoids, peels, lasers, sclerotherapy injections, and light sources. Light glycolic acid peels are often used in conjunction with antibiotics to control rosacea. A series of peels are performed every two to four weeks along with a skin care program with a low concentration of glycolic acid can be effective.

Tiny thread veins called 'telangiectasias' can be effectively zapped with lasers that emit specific wavelengths of light that target the visible blood vessels just under the skin. Heat from the laser's energy builds in the vessels, causing them to collapse. More than one treatment may be needed. With the most advanced lasers and light devices, there is little or no bruising. Intense pulsed light sources are often used to reduce redness. Once you've zapped the existing blood vessels, you will need additional treatments for new ones as they crop up. Sun will exposure cause more of them.

BEAUTY BYTES:
If you think you might have rosacea, check out www.rosacea.org.

Lasers also work for rhinophyma, a severe stage of rosacea that causes the tip of the nose to swell and the skin to become thickened and bulbous. This is much more common in men.

operation avoidance

There is a definite distinction between rosacea and run-of-the-mill sensitive skin. If you have rosacea, your skin might be sensitive and reactive.

Conquering rosacea means avoiding anything that brings on an attack. Culprits vary from person to person. Wash thoroughly with a soap-free cleanser and lukewarm water to prevent fungal infections. Medications kill bacteria, creating new space for fungi to grow. Metronidazole (in the form of Metrogel or Noritate) is commonly prescribed, as are many retinoids like Differin and others.

Things to avoid:

Lifestyle	Sun exposure • Cold and wind • Saunas, hot tubs, and steamy showers • Getting overheated • Coughing or straining • Loofahs, sponges, washcloths, and abrasives • Smoking
Skin care ingredients	Alcohol • Fragrance • Menthol • Witch hazel • Peppermint oil • Detergents • Acids • Chemical sunscreens • Astringents
Diet	Hot caffeinated drinks (tea, coffee, hot chocolate) • Foods high in niacin (liver, yeast) • Foods containing histamines (tomatoes, aubergine, cheese) • Spices (paprika, chilli, cayenne, Asian mustard) • Alcoholic beverages (wine, beer, liquor)

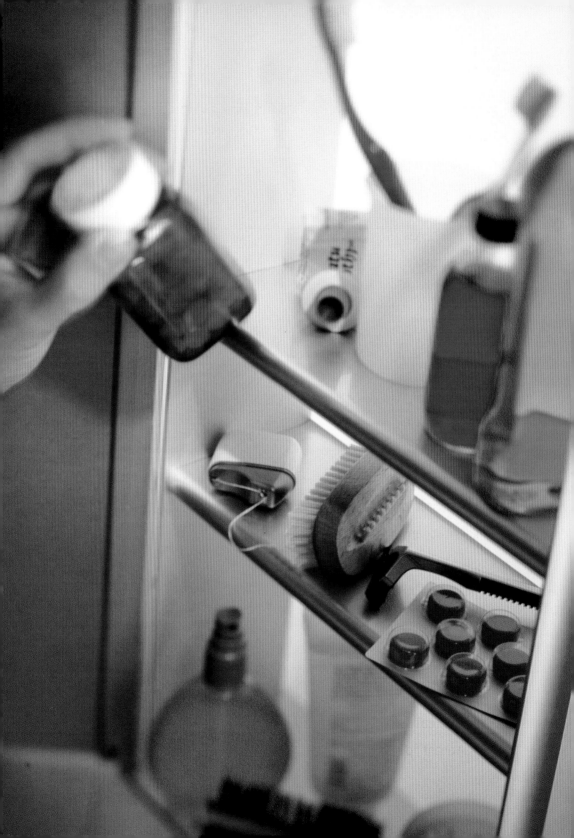

AT THE DOCTOR

With acne, there comes a time when only prescription medicines will do. With a dermatologist's help, most cases of acne can be cleared up, at least temporarily. Products available at the chemist may offer relief from some forms of acne, but won't clear up cysts lying deep within the skin or prevent new spots from appearing. If you have a chronic problem that doesn't respond, see a dermatologist. Don't let it get out of control. A doctor can treat your acne from the inside out with oral and topical medications. No one should have to suffer with acne indefinitely when there are safe and effective medications available. It may not be considered by some to be a serious medical problem but to those afflicted with spots, it can be devastating to your confidence and self esteem at any age.

Prescription medications come in a variety of forms, both topical and oral. Creams and lotions are good for older skin. Gels and solutions are best for oilier skin. All forms work to reduce sebum production and inflammation, kill bacteria and stabilise the androgen level. For breakouts in harder-to-reach areas like the back or shoulders, oral medication may be easier to use than topical antibiotics. Topical vitamin A derivatives are the cornerstone of an anti-acne treatment plan. They are often used for life in one form or another.

in the clear

in the clear

The biggest mistake women make is waiting it out. The earlier you seek treatment, the lesser chance of scarring. Antibiotics are the most common place to start.

Antibiotics are often used together with other therapies in a capsule form. It works to destroy *P. acnes* bacteria to reduce inflammation, redness and pus formation. In many cases, you will need to stay on oral antibiotics for two to four months at a time. Always finish the course unless otherwise directed by your doctor; if it is interrupted, they may become ineffective. You should follow the directions for taking your medication to the letter. Some antibiotics should be taken on an empty stomach; others are more effective when they are taken with or after meals. You might be told to take them at least one hour before bedtime. Your doctor may advise you not to take other medications or supplements – like iron or calcium – while taking some antibiotics, because they can interfere with absorption. Certain types, like the tetracyclines, are harder on the digestive tract, while others are more slowly absorbed and may have fewer side effects. If you are having trouble using the antibiotic prescribed, speak to your doctor about changing your medication. If your acne is coming back even while you are on antibiotics that were previously helpful, you may have become resistant to them. Your doctor may switch you to a different class of antibiotics. Cream, lotion and gel formulas are commonly used in addition to pills as anti-bacterial agents.
Side effects: Nausea or diarrhoea, sun sensitivity, yeast infections, headaches, dizziness, skin discolouration, tooth discolouration.

Oral antibiotics

Drug Class	Brand Name
Tetracycline	Tetracycline, Achromycin, Sumycin
Doxycycline	Doryx, Vibramycin
Minocycline	Dynacin, Minocin, Vectrin
Erythromycin	E-mycin, Ery-C, Ery-tab, E.E.S., Ery-ped, Erthrocin, PCE
Penicillin-type drugs	Ampicillin, Cephalexin
Sulfa	Bactrim, Cotrim, Septra

This is a partial list to be used as a guide. Not all drugs are available in all countries, and generic and brand names vary. Some medications that require a prescription in the UK are available over the counter in other countries. Check with your doctor or pharmacist to find out what medications are available to you.

Hormonal therapy is used to reduce the amount of androgens in a woman's body, most commonly through birth control pills. Low-dose corticosteroid drugs, such as prednisone or dexamethasone, may have an anti-inflammatory effect and suppress the androgen produced by the adrenal glands. Anti-androgen medications, such as Spironolactone, may be prescribed to help prevent androgens from causing excessive oil production.

Side effects: Menstrual irregularities, breast tenderness, headaches, fatigue.

the A list

Retinoids are derivatives of vitamin A that work to unclog pores. Retin-A has been on the market since the 1970s and is commonly used to treat wrinkles, psoriasis and acne.

Retinoids treat blackheads and whiteheads effectively and fight acne by increasing cell turnover, which helps unplug existing comedos, so other topical medications, such as antibiotics, can penetrate the follicles better. In the US and the UK, a prescription is required. In other countries, prescription-strength retinoids can be found in a pharmacy. Retinoids can dry out the skin and cause peeling and irritation. Occasionally the acne worsens during the first month of treatment because the medication draws out spots that would not otherwise have shown up yet. These side effects usually decrease or disappear when the medication has been used for a while and your skin is used to it. Tretinoin is an exfoliating agent or keratolytic, which makes it effective in removing the oil plugs that cause acne blemishes.

How to use retinoids:
Wait a half hour after cleansing to apply. Apply sparingly and at night. A pea-sized dab is enough for your entire face. Apply sunscreen before going out.

Newer acne formulas include Tazarotene (Tazorac), a potent synthetic retinoid, and Adapalene (Differin), a topical compound that helps decrease microcomedone formation. New compounds springing up all the time, so if yours stops working you can switch to another form.

Topical acne drugs

Types of drug	Brand Name	Form
Tazarotene	Avage, Tazorac	Cream, gel
Thromycin	ATS	Solution, gel
Erythromycin	Erycette	Pads
	Erygel	Gel
	Erymax	Solution
	Staticin	Solution
	T-Stat	Cream
Clindamycin	Cleocin T, Duac	Solution, gel, pads
Sulfacetamide	Klaron	Lotion
Sulphur	Sulfacet-R	Lotion
Metronidazole	Metrogel	Gel, cream, lotion
Adapalene	Differin	Gel, pads, cream
Tretinoin	Retin-A	Cream, gel, lotion
	Retin-A Micro	Gel
	Avita	Cream, gel
Azelaic Acid	Azelex	Cream

This is a partial list to be used as a guide. Not all drugs are available in all countries and generic and brand names vary. Some medications that require a prescription in the UK are available over the counter in other countries. Check with your doctor or pharmacist to find out what medications are available to you.

the last resort

the last resort

Isotretinoin is used as a last resort to clear up severe, cystic acne. Now available for over twenty years, Isotretinoin has been shown to be effective for 70–85 per cent of patients.

Isotretinoin, or RoAccutane, is the closest thing we have to an acne cure. It comes in 10, 20 or 40mg capsules that are taken with food once or twice daily. The average treatment period is four months and the strength and frequency is determined by your doctor. Additional treatment courses can be given for recurrences. The most likely candidate for repeat treatments is suffering from deep, painful, cystic acne that has not responded to the usual alternatives.

When all else fails, many acne sufferers turn to RoAccutane to clear their complexions. It is currently the only medication that actually shrinks the gland that produces the oily sebum found in acne. RoAccutane is a potent drug that can produce dramatic results, but it also comes with side effects and risks. Among the more serious of these are elevated blood cholesterol, lipid and triglyceride levels and abnormal liver enzymes and depression. Side effects vary and usually go away after the medication is stopped.

Careful screening and evaluation will be done before you can start taking the drug, as well as close monitoring and frequent blood tests during therapy. If you have difficulty tolerating it, your doctor may be able to reduce the dose of the drug. You will be

BEAUTY BYTES:

For more research, log on to The Acne Support Group, www.m2w3.com, or the British Association of Dermatologists, www.bad.org.uk

TOP TIP:

Carry a moisturising lip balm with shea butter or aloe vera if you are on RoAccutane, to reapply during the day and prevent lips from cracking.

instructed not to take other vitamin A derivatives while you are using this medicine, including supplements containing beta-carotene. With ANY form of retinoid therapy, there is increased sensitivity to the sun because the epidermis is thinner. Sunscreen with a minimum SPF 15 is a MUST. Sun exposure can cause severe irritation or burning and lead to hyperpigmentation and possible scarring.

Side effects: Dry eyes, dry mouth, dry skin, cracked, peeling lips, itching, nosebleeds, muscle aches, depression.

Topical Isotretinoin (Isotrex) is in use in Canada, Australia and other countries outside of the US. It is basically RoAccutane in a light protective sunscreen base and comes in gel or cream formula. The skin should be washed and dried before applying it sparingly once or twice daily, using enough medication to cover the entire affected area (face, chest or back). You will be instructed not to apply it to the eyelids or the skin at the corners of the eyes and mouth, and to avoid the angles of the nose. Severe redness and peeling are possible side effects. If the irritation is severe, you may be directed to use the medication less frequently, discontinue use temporarily or altogether. If your doctor has prescribed topical isotretinoin, any other topical acne therapies should be used with caution.

WARNING: Don't even think about getting pregnant while using RoAccutane. This drug cannot be taken during pregnancy or while breast-feeding because it can cause severe birth defects.

surface peels

surface peels

Chemical peels are used to unroof pustules and exfoliate. Exfoliation helps topical treatments to penetrate the skin better, to control acne and prevent outbreaks.

Peeling principles are based on the cells in the epidermis regenerating every month. Depending upon the type of peeling compound used and its concentration, the top layers of skin – epidermis and dermis – are scraped off. New skin cells begin to form a new top layer 24 hours after the procedure. 1–2 days later more new cells, called fibroblastic cells, become active in the dermis. These cells create new collagen fibres, which constitute the support structure of the newly generated skin. At the same time, the elastin fibres, which give the skin its flexibility, also begin to regenerate.

Light peels are typically repeated at intervals of 3–4 weeks, until the desired effect is achieved. A monthly or bimonthly maintenance programme will help keep acne under control. A skin-care regime containing retinoic or glycolic acid should be used regularly to preserve the results of the treatment.

Most peels can be performed on the face, chest and back, as well as the hands, arms and legs. Sun exposure should be avoided for at least a week following a peel and one week prior to your next peel visit. A sunscreen with an SPF 15 should be worn daily.

Superficial or 'lunchtime' peeling revitalizes the outer layers of skin for a smooth, rejuvenated appearance, and can be done on all skin types. For acne, peeling can considerably reduce the number of blemishes and can improve skin colour, transforming it from yellowish and dull to pink and clear.

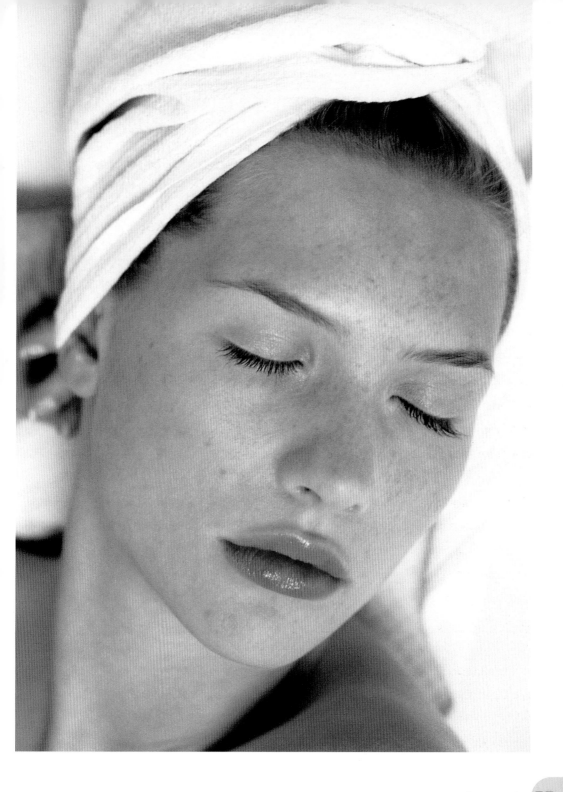

let there be light

Moving beyond the pharmacy, light-based therapies are the next wave in skin-clearing treatments.

The biggest news in acne therapy is the use of laser and light systems to destroy the bacteria that causes acne without drugs. New devices emit a narrow band spectrum of intense light directly onto the skin. When the high-intensity lamp is shined directly on the skin, it kills the bacteria. Light rays convert a substance produced by acne bacteria into an acne-killing compound. Other forms of non-invasive laser treatments deliver energy down to the oil-producing centres in the sebaceous glands to destroy these oil reservoirs without harming the outer layers of the skin. These layers may have the potential to offer a faster, more controlled treatment of severe and cystic acne, as an alternative to traditional topical or oral medicines without the side effects.

These devices may be able to achieve better results than antibiotics and destroy acne-causing bacteria for months after a single treatment. Treatments can take from 8–15 minutes and may be repeated as needed, once or twice per week for up to 8 weeks. In many cases, acne can be controlled for several months at a time. Another benefit is that results may be seen after one treatment instead of 8–12 weeks with medications. Light therapy can also speed up the healing of active lesions, reduce inflammation and improve or prevent acne scars.

Lasers and light devices used with photodynamic therapy using aminolevulinic acid for shorter treatment periods of 1 hour are also proving to be effective for acne as well as rosacea. Treatment begins with a light microdermabrasion to remove dead skin cells on the surface of the face.

Microdermabrasion is a state-of-the-art peel technique that uses a combination of force plus suction to deliver finely ground aluminium oxide or sodium crystals to smooth the skin's texture. This treatment is often combined with other acne-fighting therapies. Sloughing the epidermis allows for better penetration of the aminolevulinic acid. The medication is left on for 30–60 minutes, removed with soap and water, and then the laser or light source therapy is used.

BEAUTY BYTES:

For more information about light therapy, log on to

www.asds-net.org

wrinkles and acne

wrinkles and acne

As if puberty wasn't tough enough, what do you do when you can't decide whether wrinkles or blemishes are your biggest skin care concern?

You've got crow's-feet and frown lines, as well as spots on your cheeks, chin and forehead. While the demand for antiwrinkle products increases steadily, women also have an insatiable appetite for new and improved acne therapies. Regrettably, adult acne is more common in women than men. Women over 40 often respond well to oral antibiotics, like tetracycline, doxycycline or minocycline, as well as milder retinoids like Retin-A Micro and Avita. Newer, gentler topical acne formulas are more cosmetically elegant, making them ideal for mature skin. They can be worn discreetly under foundation without some of the redness and irritation you may have experienced earlier. Cream formulas are used more frequently than gels, which are reserved for oilier skin types. If you were treated with RoAccutane in your teens and 20s, another course may be recommended to clear up your skin now.

Skin has a pH balance of 5.5. If you're mistreating your skin by using harsh detergents, over-cleansing, over-scrubbing or layering on acids, your pH may climb to 7.5 or higher. Healthy skin will bounce back quickly, but if your skin is under siege, it can take longer to recover, leaving it more susceptible to stress. A normal pH of 5.5 protects skin from bacteria, which tend to thrive in a more alkaline environment. It is important to keep the skin moisturised while treating breakouts. The areas of the face that contain the fewest oil glands, like around the eyes and the neck, need hydration. Use a non-comedogenic moisturiser for dry areas.

For mature skins suffering from lines and lesions, the name of the game is gentle exfoliation. In these cases, mild forms of vitamin A like a low dose of prescription-strength tretinoin or over-the-counter retinols are ideal. They can work within the skin's surface where wrinkles start. Combined with a gentle formula of AHAs and BHAs, you can keep pores clean and keep future breakouts at bay. If your breakouts are chronic or severe, do not delay seeing a dermatologist to design a prescription programme that can effectively reduce oil production, fight bacterial infection and jump-start your rate of cell renewal.

If you get occasional breakouts but more often during warmer months or in humid weather, adjust your skin care routine. The challenge in treating wrinkle- and acne-prone skin is to control breakouts and keep pores clear and refined, while keeping skin hydrated and supple.

Get oil under control by targeting spot-prone areas. Then keep drier, wrinkle-prone areas, like around the eyes, neck, and upper lip, well nourished by adding light moisturising products. Trade in heavy wrinkle creams for oil-free lotions, foundations and sunscreens. Add a BHA-based gel or lotion, and use tea tree oil or benzoyl peroxide spot treatment to dab on several times a day over or under make-up that can reduce redness and zap zits fast.

EXPERT ADVICE:
You may think you have acne when it is another skin condition entirely. Perioral dermatitis can show up on the chin as little blisters.

skin care questions

Keep a journal of your acne history – what worked and what didn't, when your acne seems to flare up and potential causes. A dermatologist will evaluate the severity of your acne and suggest the therapy that they have had the most success with in treating other cases similar to yours.

Questions you should ask your doctor:

- Are there better medications to clear up my acne than the ones I've tried?

- How long will it take for my acne to clear up?

- How often should I wash the affected area?

- What is the next step if this method doesn't work effectively?

- What is the best combination of medications for my type of acne?

- What cosmetic and skin care ingredients should I avoid?

- Which salon treatments will help?

- What else can I do to help clear up my acne?

Questions your doctor might ask you:

- How long have you had acne?

- What skin products are you now using and have you used in the past?

- What medications are you currently taking?

- When do flare-ups most often occur?

- In what areas on your body and face do you have blemishes?

- Have you seen other doctors about it before?

- What treatments have you already tried?

- Did any of the treatments work? If so, which ones?

- Did your parents have acne when they were young?

- If so, how severe was their acne?

- Do you have a history of any hormonal imbalances?

- If so, what are your symptoms?

- How active are you and how much sun exposure do you get?

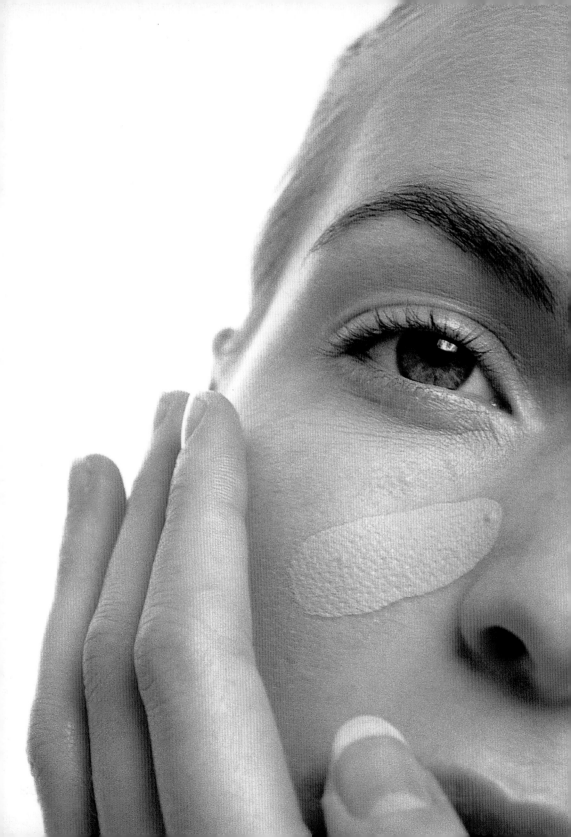

SCAR WARS

SCAR WARS

Old acne scars from your turbulent teens can ruin an otherwise smooth complexion at any age. The best way to prevent scars is to treat acne early, and for as long as necessary. Left untreated, acne can cause significant scarring that will be much more difficult to treat later on. Scars are the visible reminders of injury and tissue repair. With acne, the injury is caused by the body's inflammatory response to sebum, bacteria and dead cells in the plugged follicle. One of the main causes of scarring and delayed healing is skin fragility.

The marking of the skin frequently results from severe inflammatory cystic acne that occurs deep in the skin, and can also arise from more superficial spots. Some women bear their acne scars for a lifetime. In others, the skin undergoes some degree of remodelling and blemishes diminish in size with time. It is difficult to predict who will scar, how extensive or deep scars will be, how long they will persist and how successfully scars can be stopped from forming. The more inflammation can be prevented, the more likely it is that scarring can be avoided. Darker skin types are typically more prone to post-inflammatory hyperpigmentation, which can result in discolouration and blotchiness that lingers.

big squeeze

Keeping your hands off your face serves two purposes. It prevents the spread of bacteria that cause bad skin and helps you resist the temptation to squeeze, which causes scarring.

Squeezing forces infected material deeper into the skin, causing additional inflammation that takes longer to heal. Picking spots will not clear them up and may leave permanent scars. Tissue injured by squeezing can become infected by bacteria. Squeezing blackheads can also injure the sebaceous follicle and tissue around it, and force it deeper as well as extruding it to the skin's surface. The result can be an inflammatory reaction. Left on their own, blackheads do not usually get inflamed. Never squeeze your skin hard enough to leave an imprint. Using your fingernails can strip away pigmented cells from the deep layer of the skin and leave you with an uneven skin tone.

Picking whiteheads is potentially more harmful because they are likely to become inflamed. Microcomedos are almost too small to be seen, but you can feel them as roughness on the skin. Once they become inflamed, they may develop into a pustule or a papule. Squeezing a microcomedo or closed comedo (whitehead) will not remove the contents anyway. A microcomedo is an undeveloped comedo, so there is really nothing there to squeeze out. A whitehead has such a small follicular opening that it is nearly invisible, so no contents can be extruded. True cysts are nodules that rest deep below the surface, so you can't get to them by squeezing. Any attempt to manipulate them will just aggravate the inflammatory process. If you've got cysts, the only effective therapy comes in a pill form, usually RoAccutane.

saving face

If your complexion is being punished by unsightly brown patches that never seem to go away, you may have melasma or post inflammatory hyperpigmentation (PIH).

Skin inflammation from allergic reactions, facial waxing (especially above the lip) or spots can trigger hyperpigmentation. Sun exposure is the big culprit. Pigment may be located in the epidermis or skin's outer layer, the dermis or deeper layer, or a combination of both. The more superficial, the easier it will lighten. PIH that is more recent responds better to treatment.

Hydroquinone is the most effective skin lightening agent, but is only available in the UK in 2 per cent strength. Agents like kojic acid are often combined with azelaic acid, glycolic acids, lactic acid, retinol, ascorbic acid and botanical lighteners such as liquorice and bearberry extracts. Most skin lightening ingredients work better in tandem than on their own.

Skin lightening is not a quick process. It can take 6–12 weeks to see results. Non-prescription lightening creams can go only so far. For more dramatic improvement, look to more invasive remedies like peels and lasers to blend darkened areas. Microdermbrasion can remove superficial pigmented cells and allow lightening creams to penetrate better. Devices such as the pulse dye laser, Q-switched ruby and Nd:Yag can reduce brown coloured pigment. These systems utilise bursts of energy to target pigmented areas and destroy pigment cells. Minimising sun exposure prevents darkening of existing patches, as well as new areas. Once you have successfully lightened areas, maintenance is needed for the long term.

under cover

under cover

Cosmetic acne is less of a problem today because of the array of non-comedogenic products on the market. Using the right foundation and powder can actually absorb excess oil.

Oil-free foundations and concealers are a must. They can be a great help with covering up swelling and redness, and actually speed up the healing process. It is difficult to apply foundation during the first few weeks of treatment when skin may be flaky, red or scaly. Don't use concealer on open lesions. Apply a tinted drying gel or lotion and let them heal. Waterproof formulas don't come off with soap and water and require more cleansing and rubbing to remove, so they are not ideal for acne-prone skin. NEVER go to bed without removing make-up completely so there is no residue left on the skin overnight. Acne scars present a marathon challenge to cover them because they are generally not flat, but either raised or sunken. Carefully placed concealer with the right primer and foundation are essential.

For depressed scars: Start with a primer so foundation will flow on smoothly. Applied with a sponge, foundation gives a flawless finish for recessed areas.

For darkened or red scars: Start with a pale concealer, and add a second coat a few shades lighter than your skin. End with concealer that matches your skin, and set each layer with pressed powder.

MAKE-UP MUST-HAVES:
Powder compact and blotting papers for emergency oil spills.

make-up manoeuvres

- Apply make-up to a face that has been cleansed and is completely dry.

- Only oil-free foundation. On older or combination skin, you can try a formula with a little oil. Use a small amount applied in five dots; on the forehead, on the tip of the nose, on each cheek and on the chin.

- Gently pat dots of concealer that matches your skin tone under the eyes, on the lids, on any broken capillaries, or on very red, blemished areas. Use a camouflage brush or cotton swab to blend. Green tints can help reduce redness. Yellow is good for correcting bluish discolourations, dark circles under the eyes, and pasty complexions.

- Use a fine, matte powder all over the face, lids and around the lips to control oil. Choose a shade that won't change the hue of your concealer. Even if you don't use foundation, powder is key to set your make-up.

- If you skip the powder phase, the foundation will mix with the natural oils in your skin and melt. Foundation contains pigment particles that are broken down during the day Reapply foundation and/or powder as needed. Avoid touching your make-up after you have applied it.

scar remedies

Total restoration of the skin to the way it looked before acne first attacked is not always possible, but the skin surface can be improved to some extent.

The most common souvenir is uneven skin texture, especially visible on the softer areas of the face like the cheeks, caused by tough scar tissue that forms both on the surface and in the deeper skin layers.

Acne erupts from the deep tissue to the surface of the skin, so the scars left behind are more complex than those from cuts and scrapes. These are three-dimensional because they go through the skin.

For depressed scars, fillers can be injected under the skin to elevate the scar and fill it in. Icepick scars show up as deep pits that look like an ice pick has been jabbed into the skin, Boxcar scars that have more angular edges,

Acne scar fillers

Form	Brand Name
Polylactic acid	New Fill
Human tissue	CosmoDerm CosmoPlast
Bovine collagen	Zyplast, Zyderm
Bovine collagen with micro particles	ArteColl
Injectable liquid silicone	Silskin Silikon 1000
Hyaluronic acid	Restylane Perlane Hylaform Hylaform Plus

and Rolling scars that look like a wavelike or smooth indentation in the skin are often treated with fillers. Any filling substance can essentially be used to treat acne scars, although the most effective tend to be more thicker and longer lasting like fat and other volume fillers.

Since acne scars come in various sizes and shapes, treatments are not limited to one method. Most acne scar treatments require that your skin is free of active acne, so if you still break out seek therapies to stop spots from erupting first. Acne scar treatment should be addressed on a case by case basis – no single treatment is right for everyone. Several remedies can be used to achieve the same results. If you have been taking RoAccutane, it will be suggested that you wait 6 months to a year before having any treatment.

Hypertrophic or raised scarring can be treated through the use of silicone sheets. Cortisone injections performed by a doctor may be effective in flattening areas of thickened scar tissue. Topical remedies that can improve the skin's surface include copper peptides which may be able to stimulate collagen production. Topical retinoic acid may be applied directly on the scars as well, in higher strengths for best results.

Hyperpigmentation is a common problem, especially in darker skin types, and can be difficult to fade out. Bleaching agents and sun protection are a required first line of defense. Many of the same treatments that are used to control acne are also used to treat the scars it leaves behind. Generally, scars located on the thicker and tougher skin of the chest and back do not respond as well to treatment as facial scars.

Peel series

AHA or BHA peels, TCA peels and microdermabrasion treatments soften superficial scarring and help to even out blotchy discoloration that often accompanies acne scars. Lighter peels will often be spaced 2–4 weeks apart for best results. These treatments are a continuum – they fight new spots from forming as well as work to fade scars – and should be combined with an aggressive at-home skin-care programme.

Ablative lasers

Lasers of various wavelengths and intensities are used to recontour scar tissue and reduce the redness around healed acne lesions. Ablative lasers can improve deep scars that remain decades after acne has run its course, and in some cases, a single treatment will achieve permanent results. Because the skin absorbs bursts of energy from the laser, there may be redness for several months. The CO_2 laser vaporizes thin layers of the skin and tightens collagen fibres, which is good for depressed acne scars. The Erbium:YAG laser produces very precise bursts of energy, which allows for the sculpting of smaller, irregular scars.

Non-ablative lasers

Non-ablative lasers soften acne scars but they work slower. The laser stimulates the body to produce more collagen under the skin. The deeper the scar, the more collagen you have to make to raise the scar up. Intense Pulsed Light sources and Pulse Dye lasers must be done in a series to improve scarring. For scars that have turned white over time, the Excimer laser has proved effective in re-pigmenting scar tissue, which is particularly useful for darker skin types more prone to hypopigmentation (skin discolouring). Combination therapy with a series of laser or light-based treatments and mechanical resurfacing like microdermabrasion can be effective on large, soft areas of the face with rolling scar tissue.

Skin surgery

Individual scars may be removed by a punch excision. The scar is excised down to the layer of fat underneath the skin; the resulting hole in the skin may be repaired with sutures or with a small skin graft. 'Subcision' is a technique in which a surgical probe is used to lift the scar tissue away from unscarred skin, to elevate the depressed scar.

Face lift

In women over 40 with acne scarring, sometimes a face-lift may be recommended to stretch out the skin which can soften some of the scars. Fillers like fat can be added to improve the deepest scars at the same time. Resurfacing with lasers and peels can be done at a later stage to further smooth the surface of the skin and even out skin tone.

TOP TIP:

The best remedy for acne scars is a combination of topical therapies plus clinical treatments

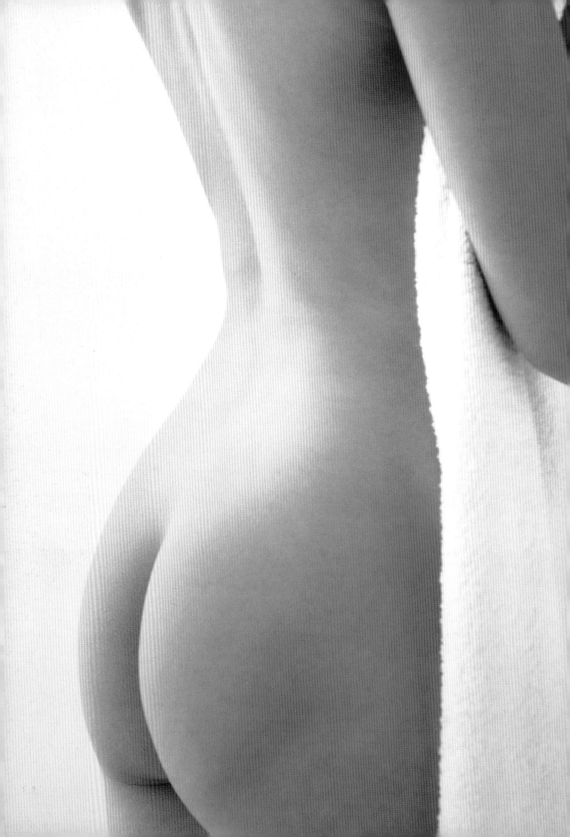

FIGURE IT OUT

For centuries, women have been at war with their fat cells. Doctors estimate that more than half of us are heavier than we should be, and about one quarter are obese. Clearly, we're eating too much and moving too little.

Losing weight isn't all that hard; the difficult part is keeping it off. All too often, our idea of a shape-up programme consists of jumping on the latest fad-diet bandwagon, which we inevitably fall off when we get bored or it stops working.

Our appetite stems from more than an empty stomach. Researchers have discovered that the urge to eat is governed largely by hormones that communicate between the tummy and the brain. If your stomach is empty, it signals the brain. One of these chemical messengers, ghrelin, is being studied for its role in stimulating the need to eat even when we are satisfied and is being looked at as a potential cure for obesity. Ghrelin levels increase during fasting and before meals, but level off after eating, and they may contribute to why some people have trouble controlling their weight long term.

In the meantime, as we already know, the safest way to lose weight is to burn off more calories than you take in. You can't lose it all in a matter of weeks. Stay away from quick fixes: they don't work.

fat fears

For many women, the fear of getting fat is a fact of life. We are about 12 per cent more likely to be obese than men, and we are far more obsessed about it.

This three-letter word is enough to instill fear in the hearts of every woman with visions of lumps, bumps, bulges and saddlebags. 90 per cent of people with eating disorders are adolescents and young women. Fashion models weigh about one-quarter less than the average female. There are some women who can consume twice as many calories as the rest of us without gaining an ounce. No one said life is fair.

Beware of diet saboteurs who tell you to reward yourself with a treat when you've lost a few pounds. If you lose the weight slowly, you'll be much more effective at keeping it off, especially if you incorporate exercise into your routine. Fat can be reduced by limiting caloric intake to a level below the energy exerted, or increasing physical activity. The bad news is that there is no magic formula that works for everyone.

Generally, an older body is a fatter body. An average 20-year-old woman's body is 16.5 per cent muscle, 47 per cent non-muscle lean tissue, 10 per cent bone and 26.5 per cent fat. By comparison, the average 20-something guy has 30 per cent muscle and only 18 per cent fat. The differences between women and men increase with age. Both sexes become fatter, but more so women.

Body fat can be measured by skinfold thickness, which is a measure of the thickness of the skin and fat lying under the skin at specific sites like the back of the upper arm. Basically, it's a scientific form of a pinch test. Another method, bioelectrical impedance analysis or BIA, sends a mild electrical current through the body, which estimates the total body water. The percentage of body water can be translated into an estimate of body fat and lean body mass. Generally, a higher per cent body water indicates a larger amount of muscle and lean tissue.

Excess fat settles in different places at different stages of life. The major culprit is oestrogen. Around the age of 40, women often find it gets harder and harder to keep the weight off. Menopause adds a layer of fat around the middle.

Teens and 20s: Any excess fat is distributed evenly around your body.
30s and 40s: Extra weight goes straight to your hips and thighs.
50s: Added pounds head for your waistline and stay put.
60s and 70s: If you have been steadily gaining weight through the years, expect to be somewhat pear-shaped.

The older you get, the harder it is to lose weight because your body settles in, gets lazy and grows accustomed to your fat. The shifting also tends to follow the pattern of gravity – it gets lower. There is a tendency for the shoulders to narrow, the chest size to grow, and the pelvis to widen over the years. Chest size in women peaks between the ages of 55 and 64. Although a bigger chest may seem like something to look forward to, it is usually accompanied by the flattening and sagging of the breasts. After age 65, a woman's chest generally shrinks. The pelvis, in contrast, keeps widening throughout life, which accounts for the pear shape period.

body mass

Body weight represents a sum of the bodily structures including muscle, bone, water and stored fat. One measure of plumpness is the dreaded Body Mass Index (BMI), which, at first glance, reads like an Einstein theory in physics.

BMI is determined by dividing your weight in kilos by your height in metres squared. For example, a woman who is 1.65m and weighs 82 kilos would have a BMI of just over 30. You are considered overweight if your BMI is 25–29.9, moderately obese if you have a BMI of 30 or more. However, not every woman fits neatly into BMI charts or height/weight statistics. If you have a large amount of muscle, which weighs more than fat, your weight may seem higher than normal limits. Lean body mass is commonly used to describe the muscles in your arms, legs, back, neck and abdomen. Body composition is your proportion of fat to muscle. A woman needs a minimum of 13–17 per cent body fat for regular menstruation. If it is lower, periods may stop and you could become infertile.

The healthy ranges of body fat are higher for women than for men, and the range increases slightly with age. Generally, a BMI of greater than 27.3 per cent for women or 27.8 per cent for men would be considered overweight.

BODY MASS INDEX

BMI = weight in kg ÷ height in m squared

eg: 1.65m x 1.65m = 2.72

82 kilos ÷ 2.72 = 30.1 BMI

just the fat

Age	Healthy range of body fat
18–39	21–32%
40–59	23–33%
60–79	24–35%

Counting fat grams is one way to get a clear picture of your daily totals. The trick is to maintain a diet of less than 30 per cent fat.

Nutritionists recommend sticking to foods that have less than 5g fat. This allows you a treat of a few higher fat foods as long as they fit within your daily limit. If you only eat foods that are 30 per cent fat or lower, your diet is guaranteed to be less than 30 per cent fat, but that can be limiting. Diets with less than 20 per cent fat leave you unsatisfied and likely to overeat when willpower crumbles. To calculate the percentage of fat in your diet, at the end of the day, add up the fat grams and total calories. Work out your daily percentage by multiplying the fat grams by 9 to get fat calories. Divide this number by the total calories. The final number should be less than 30 per cent. For example:

> Total calories for day: 1950
> Total fat grams: 36
> 36 fat grams x 9 calories per fat gram = 324 fat calories
> Fat calories (324) ÷ total calories (2069) = 16.6% of calories from fat

Invest in a body fat monitor/scale that can estimate your body fat. To get the most accurate results, avoid moderate activity for 12 hours, don't eat for 4 hours or drink alcohol for 48 hours before stepping on the scales.

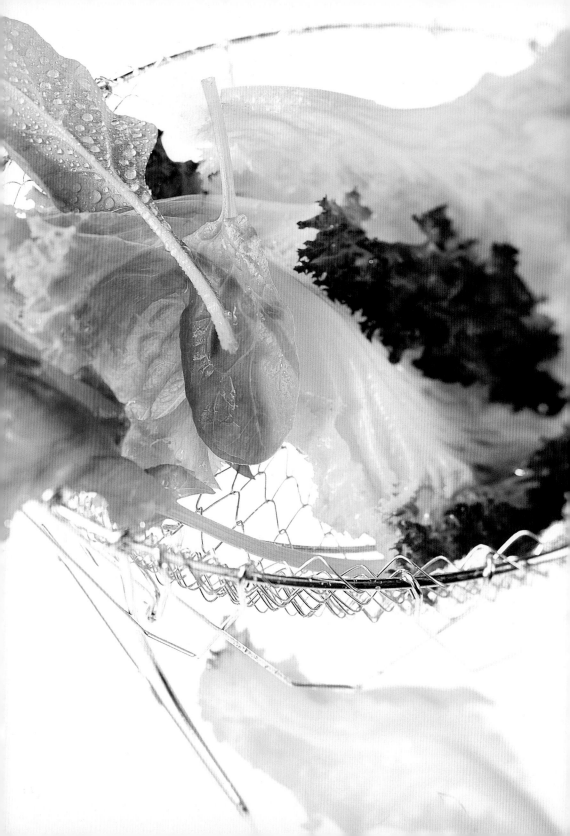

FAT FREEDOM

FAT FREEDOM

Shopping for a new 'diet' can be a daunting experience. We've all been there and done that. The average dieter often ends up heavier afterwards. Diets offer only short term solutions; they are destined to become something you go on and come off because they are so limiting. Failing at dieting can also ravage your self-esteem. It's hard to know which diet is best for you. Deciphering the merits of high protein-low carb versus high carb-low fat versus optimising your protein-carb blend, can drive you to the dessert menu. Plus no two doctors agree on any diet programme. Sometimes you lose weight best when you listen to your body, instead of adhering to a generic regime.

Decide whether you want to lose weight or maintain your weight. Consider your activity level; sedentary (total couch potato), light exercise (housework, walking up 5 flights of steps, pushing a pram), moderate exercise including aerobic activity (spinning classes, walking to work) or an active lifestyle (a few laps around the pool each day, running with the dog every morning). Determine a weight that is comfortable for you, and make it realistic. You may be better off stabilising than struggling to lose more weight. As we age, our bodies become a giant fat magnet, making our efforts that much harder as well as more vital.

tipping the scales

tipping the scales

A certified nutritionist or personal trainer makes the difference between dieting and working out day after day and not making any progress, to achieving the shape of your dreams.

Just because your trainer looks like an Olympic medalist, it doesn't necessarily mean they know anything about fitness and physiology. Check out their credentials before you sign up. Nutrition and fitness experts come with varying degrees of expertise, and many are certified in more than one area of specialisation like weight management, weight training or strength training. A registered dietitian is an expert in the science of nutrition and dietetics who is able to assist in evaluating nutritional information and supplementation, and translate it into practical application.

Determine your needs in terms of expertise, whether you are more comfortable with a man or a woman, billing, flexibility, scheduling sessions, frequency and rates. Ask for references and get referrals from satisfied people who have used trainers and nutritional counsellors. Make sure they carry liability insurance. If you're under medical care, they should request a health screening from your doctor. Look for someone who motivates you and with whom you can get along with long-term. A good place to start is at your gym. A trainer or fitness professional who works in a club will probably charge less per hour than one who works independently and comes to your home or office.

To find a qualified nutrition expert, log on to www.eatright.org, www.findanutritionist.com or www.cdc.gov/niosh/diet/dietpac.html.

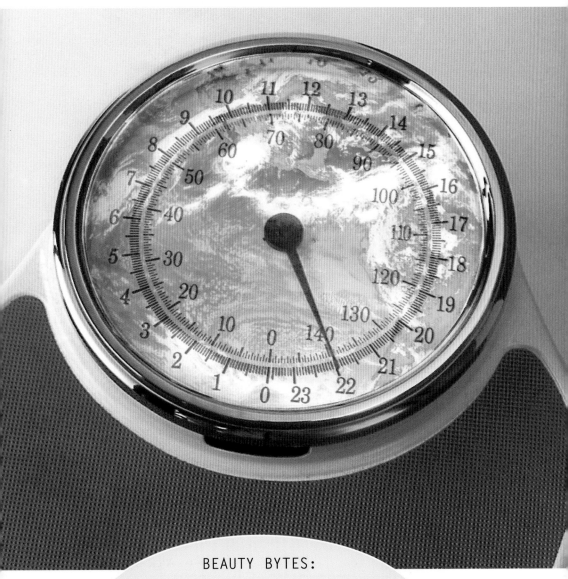

use it to lose it

use it to lose it

Exercise is the most effective treatment for fat reduction. Committing to a regular exercise programme gives you the best chance of maintaining your weight loss.

Many women look at their overweight parents and come to the conclusion: 'I'm destined to be overweight and there's nothing I can do about it.' Some of us have genes that pre-dispose us to being overweight, and some overweight people may have an impaired metabolism that makes it harder. Neither of these facts preclude you from maintaining or losing weight. Genetics accounts for only 25 per cent of your risk of becoming plump.

Take advantage of every opportunity to be active; take the stairs instead of the lift, walk instead of hailing a taxi, walk briskly instead of strolling and park at the far end of the car park so you'll have to walk an extra few metres. Try to find some extra time in your day to sneak in a 15-minute jog or a quick aerobics class. Keep workout clothes in your office or car just in case the opportunity arises. It all adds up.

REALITY CHECK:

Both weight training and cardiovascular exercise are essential. The more lean muscle tissue you have, the higher your resting metabolic rate will be. By developing more muscle, you will be burning more body fat all day long, even when you're not working out.

food diary

food diary

Sometimes putting it all on paper makes it official. Keep track of what you are consuming during the course of the day, and the week. You may be in for a shocker.

This will help focus you on where the hidden fat and calories are coming from that can sabotage your slimming programme.

Day	Breakfast	Lunch	Dinner	Snacks	Calories	Fats
Monday						
Tuesday						
Wednesday						
Thursday						
Friday						
Saturday						
Sunday						

fat busters

Don't assume that because a food is 'low fat' you can eat as much as you want. Calories count, too. So does serving size.

Fat provides 9 calories per gram, more than twice the number provided by carbohydrates or protein, and essential fatty acids, which are not made by the body and must be obtained from food. Fatty acids provide the raw materials that help in the control of blood pressure, blood clotting, inflammation and other bodily functions, and are the primary components of dietary fats. Omega-3 fatty acid or fish oil is a polyunsaturated fat found in fatty fish like salmon. This type of fat helps increase healthy cholesterol, decrease bad cholesterol in the blood, and may lower blood pressure by lowering triglycerides.

REALITY CHECK: Alcohol can make you feel bloated and add on the pounds. For example, a 6oz glass of chardonnay contains 90 calories whilst half a pint of lager has 150 calories.

Fat helps in the absorption of the fat-soluble vitamins A, D and E, and helps maintain the immune system. You don't want to eliminate it completely, just limit what you take in to what you need and nothing more. Stick to 'low-fat' and 'fat-free' products whenever possible, and be sceptical about labels and claims. Note the serving size used when looking at nutritional information on packets. If the serving size is 100g, if you consume 200g, remember that the amount of fat, sugar, etc. doubles too.

Reading matters

What it says	What it means
Reduced fat	25% less fat than whatever it is being compared to
Light or lite	50% less fat than whatever it is being compared to
Low-fat	One serving has fewer than 3g of fat
Fat-free	One serving has less than 0.5g of fat
Lean (meats, seafood, poultry)	Less than 10g of fat, 4.5g of saturated fat, and 95mg of cholesterol per serving and per 100g
Extra lean	Less than 5g of fat, 2g of saturated fat, and 95mg of cholesterol per serving and 100g
Cholesterol-free	Less than 2mg cholesterol and 2g or less saturated fat per serving
Low cholesterol	20mg or less cholesterol per serving and 2g or less saturated fat per serving
High fibre	5g or more fibre per serving
Sugar-free	Less than 0.5g of sugar per serving
Sodium-free	Less than 5mg sodium per serving
Low sodium	140mg or less per serving
Light (in sodium)	50% reduction in sodium

magic bullets

magic bullets

Diet supplements, fat burners and miracle pills come and go. The purpose is always the same: a cure for fat without any effort. These offer only short-term solutions.

Drugs can promote weight loss for a while, but as soon as you stop taking them, the weight will pile back on unless you change your ways. Pills cannot alter the way your body handles fat, they only make temporary adjustments.

Appetite suppressants

Medications most often used in managing obesity are 'appetite suppressants'. These drugs promote weight loss by decreasing appetite or increasing the feeling of being full. They decrease appetite by increasing serotonin or catecholamine, two brain chemicals that affect mood and hunger. Some antidepressants have also been used to this effect. These medications can lead to an average weight loss of 5 pounds to 1.5 stone above what would be expected by dieting alone. They are not recommended for someone who is mildly overweight or has less than a stone to lose.

Maximum weight loss usually occurs within the first 6 months, and then tends to level off. Most appetite suppressants are recommended only for short-term use – a few weeks to a few months – and not for more than one year continuously. Sibutramine (Meridia) has been banned in some countries due to the risk of high blood pressure. Find out about potential risks like irritability, sleeplessness, nervousness, dizziness and elevations in blood pressure and pulse. Sometimes it is recommended to take the last dose during the afternoon to avoid trouble sleeping at night.

All prescription diet medications are 'controlled substances', meaning doctors need to follow certain restrictions when prescribing them. Diet drugs are not 'magic bullets' or a one-shot fix. They won't take the place of normal dieting and exercise. Their major role is to help you jump start and stay on a diet and exercise plan. Studies have shown that the majority of people who stop taking appetite suppressant medications regain the weight they had lost. Medications should be taken only under strict medical supervision, and at the dosage directed. Buying them online and self-treating can be risky.

Fat blockers

Fat blockers are anti-obesity drugs with the ability to stop foods from turning into fat cells within the body. This class of drugs is called 'lipase inhibitors'. They differ from other weight loss drugs in that they block the breakdown and absorption of fat from the gastrointestinal tract. Because they allow fat to be excreted in the stool, there are possible side effects, such as bloating, diarrhoea, and flatulence. For example, Orlistat (Xenical) is taken 3 times a day, and you may be advised to take a supplement rich in the fat-soluble vitamins A, D, E and K, and to curtail their fat intake. While taking these drugs, if you eat high-fat foods, the side effects increase. If you eat a meal that contains no fat or skip a meal, a dose of medication may be skipped.

get thin quick

If it sounds too good to be true, it is, especially when it comes to diets in a capsule, pill or teacup. Supplements alone will never get you svelte. You have to do your part.

We've all read the tempting claims; tablets that burn fat before food is digested, pills that help you go down two dress sizes without dieting or exercise, and products that burn body fat while you sleep. The list of 'natural' diet aids includes vitamins, minerals, herbs, botanicals, teas and other plant-derived substances, amino acids and concentrates, metabolites, constituents, and extracts of these substances. Their general mode of action is to burn fat by increasing the basal metabolic rate, which translates to burning more calories. Other products work by enhancing your energy levels, assisting with digestion, reducing your appetite and easing water retention.

Nutritional supplements are not required to undergo the rigorous testing that a drug is subjected to, so manufacturers do not have to demonstrate that their product is either safe or effective. As a result, little is known about potential drug interactions, dosages and long-term effects. Some of these potent ingredients can increase your blood pressure, interfere with the heart's normal rhythm, or cause strokes. Other side effects include nervousness, anxiety and

BEAUTY BYTE:

Beware of diet saboteurs who urge you to sway from your regime as a treat.

insomnia. Among the most popular fat-loss formulas, caffeine-based supplements have been linked with heart attacks and strokes, and kava kava has been cited as causing liver damage. Deaths, heart attacks and seizures have been reported from the use of Ephedra, the Chinese herb ma huang, contained in many so-called 'natural' diet remedies.

BEAUTY BYTE:
To find out more about dietary supplements, log on to www.ific.org or www.faseb.org.

Other ingredients have been touted as speeding up the metabolism, but most of these have little or no clinical data to support the claims. Pyruvate, a naturally occuring enzyme, is supposed to speed up the metabolism, chromium picolinate in capsules and tablet form is cited for regulating insulin intake but does not work for weight loss. Laxative abuse can cause dangerously low potassium levels, arrhythmia and damage to the pancreas.

Supplements are products taken by mouth that contain a 'dietary ingredient' in many forms such as tablets, capsules, soft gels, gelcaps, liquids, powders, or bars. Manufacturers may make three types of claims: health, structure or function, and nutritional content. However, there are no regulations limiting serving size or the quantity of any nutrient.

The term 'natural' does not guarantee that any product is safe. Look for ingredients in products with the U.S.P. notation, which indicates the manufacturer followed US Pharmacopoeia guidelines. Consider the name of the manufacturer or distributor; supplements made by a nationally known food and drug manufacturer are more likely to be safe.

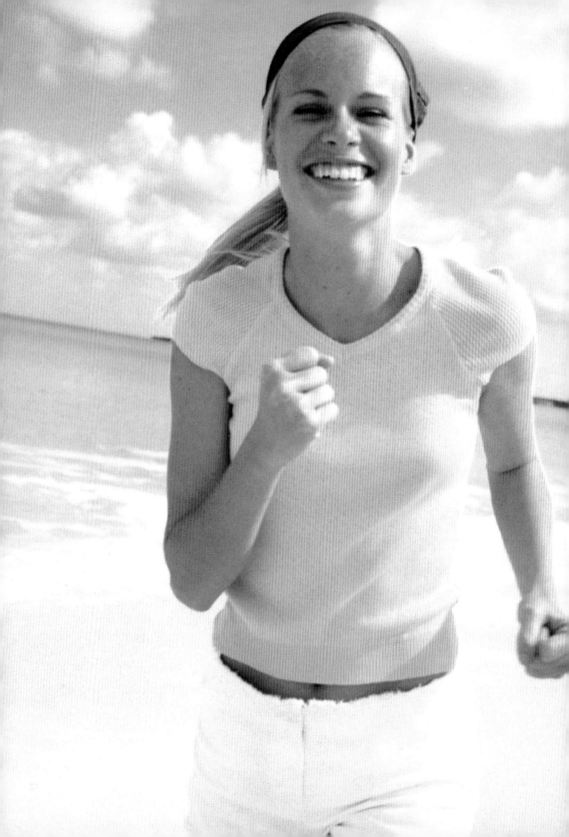

GET MOVING

GET MOVING

It should come as no surprise that from your 20s, muscle mass and metabolism decline. You can't eat the same way in your 40s and stay trim. Activity levels also tend to decrease with age. If you have a slow metabolism to start with, it becomes harder to maintain your size as you get older. Add pregnancy and hormonal changes, and it takes a concentrated effort to avoid piling on the pounds. As you age, you have to eat less and increase your activity levels.

If you've been inactive for a while, don't despair. Muscles don't go to mush overnight. Skip a week of exercise and you won't see much difference in your overall ability or strength. Miss a month and you can expect to huff and puff a little more when you restart. Skip 3 months and your body may need retraining. Take 6 months off and you'll be in the same cardiovascular shape as before you first started exercising.

When you start any new form of training, your body will improve. Vary the intensity and duration of your workouts and type of activities you do for consistently good results. Use the correct technique and learn a few different ways to exercise each muscle group in case you can't get to the machine you want at the gym. Choose exercises that simultaneously work several major muscle groups. Your equipment or gym should be accessible and convenient. Working out becomes a chore if you have to drive to the healthclub every time you want to pump some iron.

body image

Loathing your body can prevent you from living a happy, normal life. For some, how you think you look can be crippling.

Many women look in the mirror every day and hate what they see. They worry incessantly about their weight and appearance, and may become obsessed with a perceived defect. They have a very distorted view of how they look, and it does not match how others see them. Body dysmorphic disorder (BDD), a type of anxiety disorder, is a growing concern. Some BDD sufferers are able to function and cope with daily life, but others experience paralyzing symptoms of depression and anxiety. This condition is thought to be associated with a chemical imbalance in the brain which may be genetically based.

The signs vary and may include comparing the appearance of the perceived defect with that of others, frequently examining the appearance of the specific body part, camouflaging the perceived defect, attempting to convince others that it is unattractive, avoiding looking into mirrors, constantly touching the area and paralysing feelings of self-consciousness.

REALITY CHECK:
Don't be embarrassed to see your GP for a referal to a qualified specialist for treatment. For more information on eating and body image disorders, log onto: www.edauk.com, www.mentalhealth.org.uk, www.babcp.org.uk.

fat obsession

Every woman worries about her shape, but being consumed by it can lead to eating disorders and obsessions about your body.

Eating disorders are on the rise, especially among young girls and middle-aged women. Estimates are that between 5–20 per cent of sufferers die as a result of complications including metabolic and gastrointestinal problems, arrhythmia and, in extreme cases, suicide. The earlier you seek help, the better your chance of a full recovery. Eating disorders are not a sign of a problem with food, rather they are symptoms of underlying psychological and emotional problems.

Compulsive eating behaviour manifests itself in several forms; bulimia nervosa, binge eating and compulsive eating. Bulimics purge by vomiting or using laxatives – some actually binge and purge several times a day. Anorexics restrict their food intake to a range that is considered far below normal. A newer disorder is known as exercise bulimia, in which sufferers work out for many hours every day to burn a high number of calories. The classic sign is a super slim woman constantly complains about how big her thighs are. Causes of eating disorders include genetics, obesity, depression, substance abuse, yo-yo dieting and certain activities like gymnastics and ballet. Eating disorders can be tricky to spot. Most sufferers are adept at hiding their behaviour from even their closest friends and family. Treatment involves working to help restore a positive body image. Some people think that cosmetic surgery is the answer – but that can often make matters worse. The problem is really in your mind and having liposuction to reduce the size of your already thin thighs will not improve your mental state.

post-pregnancy shape-up

We can't all look like a celebrity mum a few months after childbirth, but developing a pre- and post-pregnancy plan can get your body back in shape faster.

If you start out in top physical condition with strong abdominal muscles, recovery after pregnancy will be easier. Weakening of the pelvic floor, the muscles that support your bladder and bowel, is common after childbirth. Effects include a tendency to leak, especially when you jump, cough or sneeze. Hormonal changes during pregnancy relax these muscles, and their tightness doesn't always return. Start pelvic floor exercises as soon as possible after the birth.

The old rules of diet and exercise sometimes don't work once you give birth. Most women find that with each child, the extra pounds are harder to take off. If you don't lose them during the first 4–6 months, they may never come off. This is especially true for women who gain more than 2 stone, and becomes even harder after multiple pregnancies. It is not easy to exercise or eat right when you have little ones to look after. Sleep deprivation is a problem and postnatal depression can make it more difficult. If you are breastfeeding, you cannot diet because you have to meet the nutritional requirements to produce healthy milk for your baby.

Wait until your post-natal check-up with your doctor before you start vigorous exercise classes or resuming your routine. If you've had a Caesarian section, you may be instructed to wait 6 weeks or longer. Resume your programme gradually, allowing your stamina and strength to return as you progress. Don't despair – it will take time to get back to your pre-baby shape. but it can be done. It seems only fair that after 2 or 3 babies every woman should get a certificate to a cosmetic surgeon, since every part of your body will have changed. If you are a new mum considering a cosmetic overhaul, wait a minimum of 6–9 months after childbirth or until you have finished breastfeeding. Your body needs this period to adjust and stabilise, and you need time to get used to your new lifestyle.

As the pelvis area expands during pregnancy, women take on a more 'squared-off' shape. The contour of the lower abdomen, upper thighs and hips also tends to spread. Although it is tempting to turn to liposuction to reduce any girth that is resistant to diet and exercise, losing as much of your pregnancy weight on your own is always the best course of action.

BEAUTY BYTES:
For help with post-pregnancy weight loss, go to www.weightlossresources.co.uk or www.nutricise.com
For information about cosmetic surgery, visit www.wlbeauty.com or www.surgery.org

Breast implants are an option for women who were small breasted and have lost whatever volume they had after breastfeeding. Women who breastfeed commonly complain that the shape of their breasts becomes droopier. Put off the decision to have more invasive procedures like a tummy tuck, breast lift or reduction until you have finished having children. These procedures involve skin removal and tightening. Going through another pregnancy afterwards will stretch out the thin skin again. You also may not want to be away from your baby during the prolonged recovery period.

stretch mark survival

Stretch marks can appear anywhere on the body where the skin has been stretched – like breasts, thighs, buttocks and abdomen. Advances in laser technology can reduce the pigment in stretchmarks so thay they fade away faster.

Stretch marks occur in the dermis, which makes them more difficult to treat than if they appeared on the surface on the skin. When the dermis is constantly stretched over time, the skin loses elasticity and the connective fibres break. Depending on your natural skin colouring, they may start out as raised pink, reddish brown or dark brown striations that then turn a deeper violet or purple. Over time, the marks flatten and fade to a colour a few shades lighter than your natural skin tone, white or pink, and take on a translucent quality.

Laser treatment with IPLs and non-ablative lasers target the pigment in the skin to fade and flatten them. A series of multiple treatments will be required for visible results. Laser therapy is often combined with aggressive microdermabrasion and topical remedies including retinoic acid to strengthen the dermal layer, and AHAs to exfoliate the skin's surface.

Start treatment early. Mature or pale, flesh-coloured marks do not respond as well to treatment. However, repigmenting lasers can now be used to restore pigment to lighter stretch marks.

BEAUTY BYTES:

For advice on dealing with stretchmarks, log on to:

www.wlbeauty.com

you're so vein

you're so vein

Thread veins or spider veins lie close to the surface of the skin and appear as small clusters of red, blue or purple veins that show up on the thighs, calves and ankles. The treatments are injections and lasers.

You cannot prevent thread veins entirely. Many factors are cited as the cause, including heredity, pregnancy, hormonal shifts, weight gain, prolonged sitting or standing and wearing high heels. The most common procedure calls for the veins to be injected with a saline solution, which causes them to collapse and then fade, called sclerotherapy. After each session, the veins will appear lighter. Lasers are also used to target the vessels and shrink them.

The veins worked on will be gone permanently, but new ones may appear in the future, especially if you are prone to getting them. Treatments need to be repeated, depending on the severity and the number of veins. Tight-fitting support hose are worn to guard against blood clots for 72 hours or longer. You may notice bruising and reddish areas at the injection sites or where the laser has zapped the veins. In some cases, a residual brownish pigmentation may take up to a year to fade.

Varicose veins differ from spider veins in that they tend to bulge and are larger and darker in colour. Sclerotherapy may be used to treat varicose veins but usually surgical treatment is necessary. A hand-held Doppler ultrasound device may be used to detect signs of more serious deep vein problems.

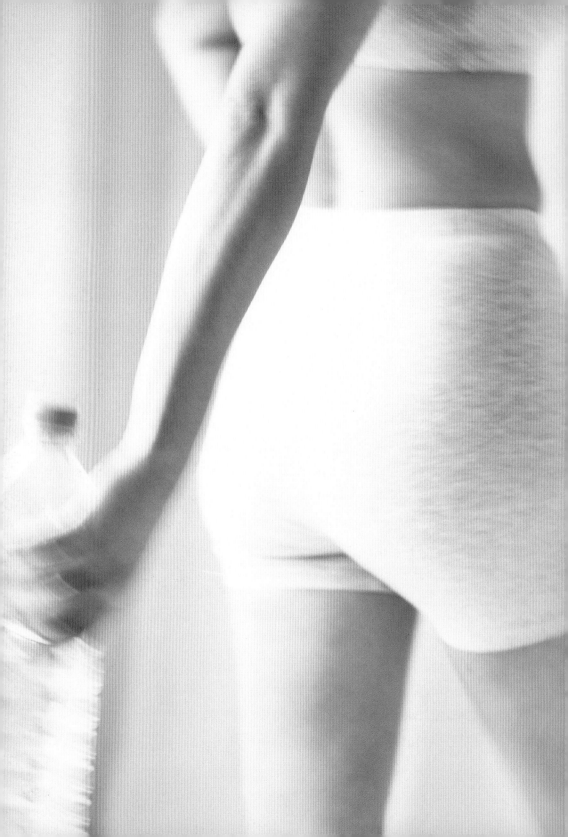

THE WAR ON DIMPLES

THE WAR ON DIMPLES

What does every woman over 20 have behind her? Cellulite. An estimated 80-90 per cent of women have some form of cellulite. The many causes begin with the usual suspects like genetics, stress, hormonal shifts, nutrition and smoking, and include excess fat, crash dieting, processed foods in the diet, a sedentary lifestyle and rapid weight gain.

Cellulite lives in the subcutaneous layer of the skin. There is a hormonal component, which explains why men don't get it. It varies in thickness and is laced with fat cells held in place by a network of fibres that cushions the muscles and organs. As we mature, the outer layer of the skin thins so the dimples become more obvious. The most cellulite-prone areas are the buttocks and thighs. Some topical creams, deep-tissue massage and ultrasound may offer temporary improvement, but there is no scientifically proven treatment that gets rid of it permanently. The best bet is a lifestyle approach, but it takes work.

A major contributing factor to the controversy surrounding solutions for lumps and bumps is that there has been no standardised means of measuring cellulite, making it difficult to gauge whether improvements have indeed occurred. In fact, some doctors to this day still deny that cellulite is any other than garden variety fat.

the bottom line

the bottom line

Cellulite is not a factor of body weight. All women know that you don't have to be plump to have cellulite. Even thin women have it.

Cellulite is not a new concept – we have just become more focused on it in recent years. It can affect any woman, regardless of size, weight and body type. At some point, whether you're a size 6 or 16, if you're female, you're likely to see a skin pattern developing that looks a bit like quilting – and I don't mean the kind on Chanel bags. It starts on the back of your thighs, extends to the buttocks and eventually travels to the dreaded saddlebags, the fronts of the thighs, buttocks, knees and upper abdomen. This is cellulite, the lumpy, bumpy bits that have been known to reduce grown women to tears.

Oestrogen production makes cellulite unique to women. Taking oral contraceptives has been cited as a possible cause. Any fluctuation in hormone levels contributes to fat storage in the fat cells. As they expand to make room for extra fat, connective fibres are pulled down and fat cells bulge out. The skin is connected to the underlying structures by vertical fibrous bands,

TWO TYPES
OF CELLULITE:
1. Dimples you see only
when you squeeze.
2. Dimples you can
see all the time.

which act like buttons on a mattress, blocking the drainage of lymph fluid. As the trapped lymph fluid collects, the fibres get tighter and these areas of skin balloon up, causing dimpling. All of these factors create the dreaded 'orange peel' and 'cottage cheese' effect.

Changing your habits is the key to the long-term management of cellulite. The fact is that most of us are simply not willing to make the lifelong commitment. The good news is that even making small changes will offer some benefits. Eating whole pure foods, eliminating alcohol and nicotine, and increasing aerobic exercise will help. While dieting alone won't get rid of lumps and bumps, burning fat and toning muscles will improve the look of them.

eating patterns

eating patterns

A good way to fight cellulite is by watching what you eat. Add foods that are easy for the body to break down, use and get rid of, and subtract anything that inhibits that process.

Drink 2–3 litres of water a day to assist your body in getting rid of unwanted toxins and waste. Be good to your liver so it will metabolize fats more efficiently and you'll be less likely to develop the dreaded 'C' word.

DOs Fresh fruits • Raw vegetables • Whole-grain foods • Low fat • High fibre • Complex carbohydrates • Water

DON'Ts Chocolate • Caffeine • Fizzy drinks • Alcohol • Sugar • Starches • Salt • Spices • Animal fats • Dairy • White flour • Processed foods • Fried foods

Some foods that may help in your battle against cellulite include natural substances like juniper berries, kelp, salmon oil, ginger, onion, pepper, fennel and orange. Seasonings may include rosemary, cayenne, cloves and cinnamon. Supplements containing lecithin, linoleic acid, flaxseed, coenzyme Q10 and glucosamine have been cited to help.

TOP TIP:
Avoid the 'ine's' – caffeine, nicotine, wine, saccharine, margarine, and theobromine (chocolate).

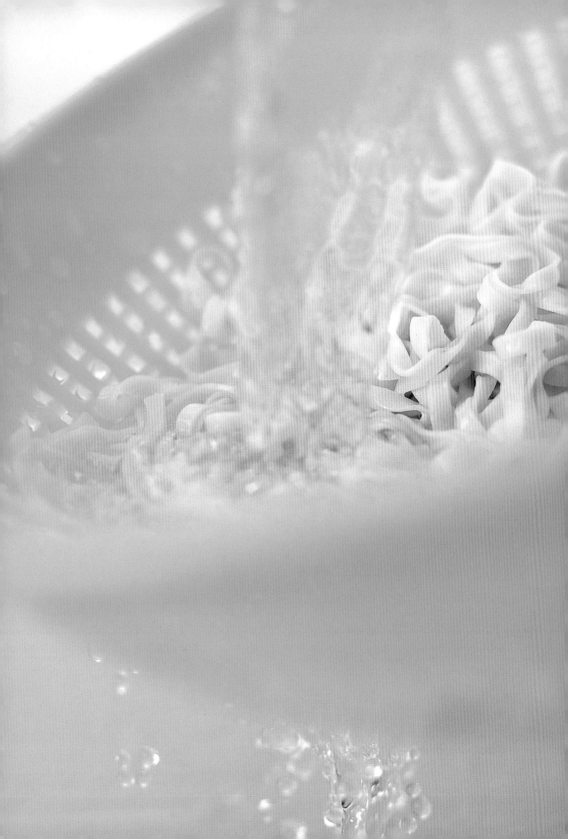

heavenly bodies

Cellulite may seem more ominous than regular fat but it is just arranged differently. Weight loss and exercise will help minimise it but you can still have lumps and bumps.

Kneading me

Massage techniques increase the circulation of blood and flow of lymph, a milky white fluid that carries impurities and waste out of the tissues. The oxygen capacity of the blood can increase by as much as 10–15 per cent after vigorous massage. By manipulating the muscles, therapeutic massage stimulates the circulatory and lymphatic systems that break down fatty tissue. The lymph fluid does not circulate throughout the body as blood does, so it has to be moved around by putting pressure on the muscles so they contract. When you are still, the muscles contract less and consequently fail to stimulate lymph flow on their own.

The Swiss method of manual lymphatic drainage has an instant, but temporary, slimming effect. This technique can be used all over the body, from the face and neck down to the ankles, where fluid tends to settle. Deep tissue massage can also be useful by targeting areas that are difficult to stimulate with exercise, such as the inner knee and upper thigh. Simply massaging each leg in circular movements for a couple of minutes each day can help get your blood flowing.

Skin-fold rolling

Endermologie, the skin-fold rolling

BEAUTY BYTE:
For more about massage techniques visit
www.amtamassage.org.

technology developed in France, temporarily reduces the appearance of cellulite. The operative word is 'temporarily'. Endermologie works by causing a swelling to the skin and underlying layers, which flattens out lumps and bumps. It is not the total answer; it is part of a multi-pronged approach to slimming and toning. A suction-roller device smooths the skin surface and stimulates circulation by eliminating toxins in the tissues.

Before the treatment, you slip into a sheer, white nylon leotard that runs from your neck to your ankles. Once you see yourself in this body stocking, you are sure to sign on for lifetime membership. Treatment begins with the therapist working on the back, then the calves, buttocks, thighs, feet, backs of the arms, and on to the neck and face. After a series of forty-minute sessions once or twice per week for four to five months, be prepared for monthly maintenance or you can kiss your progress good-bye. Endermologie doesn't take away excess fat or any dress sizes. It works well as an adjunct to body liposuction to smooth and tone the skin once the fat cells are removed and has been shown to speed up the healing process.

Thalassotherapy

Original thalassotherapy involves the use of seawater and sea air pumped from the ocean. Spa treatments are designed to recreate the benefits of the thalassotherapy experience. Ocean-derived ingredients include seaweed, sea minerals, and sea mud. Seaweed and algae saturated with mineral salts, trace elements, and amino acids are known for their rejuvenative properties and have long been used for weight loss and many ailments. With the properties of human plasma, seaweed absorbs nutrients of the sea, which transfer to the body when placed on the skin. Seaweeds are excellent sources of several vitamins, pantothenic acid, folic acid, niacin, and iodine. They are rich in minerals, especially potassium, calcium, magnesium, phosphorus, iron, zinc, and manganese. The treatments help encourage the body to eliminate waste materials, reduce excess water retention, and improve circulation.

Shrink wrap

Body wraps are commonly found on the menu of spa treatments for invigorating and detoxifying the skin. The body is usually swathed for up to an hour in mineral-rich mud, herbs, and/or seaweed-soaked cloths that aid in circulation and work to firm body contours. You can expect to be wrapped from your chest to your toes and even your arms while lying on a thermal blanket to keep you warm and cozy. A technician then unwraps you and for the finishing touch, a body massage may be done to enhance circulation and encourage oxygen to flow to blocked tissues.

Dry brushing

Dry skin brushing is used to remove dried, dead cells that block the pores of the skin to allow the skin to breathe more easily and increase its ability to protect and eliminate the waste produced by metabolism. Dry brushing can also improve the skin's texture and appearance. It should be done using a natural-bristle body brush, a horsehair or nylon bristle brush, or a glove, before taking a bath or shower. Start with the lower limbs, arms, and back, then the front of the body, brushing the skin in an upward movement towards the heart, using a moderate pressure and short strokes. The face can be done as well, using a soft brush in circular motions. Dry brushing stimulates and increases blood circulation in all organs and tissues, especially capillaries near the skin. It aids the skin in ridding the system of toxins, placing less of a burden on the organs and nerve endings in the skin.

Mesotherapy

The technique of Mesotherapy was developed by Dr Pistor in 1958 in France, to stimulate the mesoderm, or middle layer of the skin, using injections. The fibrous connective tissues, cartilage, bone, muscle and fat make up the mesoderm layer. Natural plant extracts are used with a combination of agents like enzymes and nutrients to stimulate venous and lymph flow. Some doctors use a solution containing a vasodilator, which increases blood flow and stimulates lymph drainage, and a lipolytic agent to break down fat tissue. An anaesthetic may also be used. Mesotherapy injections are given to improve the venous and lymphatic flow and also to break down the fat nodules. Extremely small needles are used, which just penetrate the body superficially, typically 4–6 millimetres. The treatments are usually given once per week. As improvement is seen, the procedure may be repeated less frequently, such as once every 2 weeks or once a month. For long-term chronic conditions such as cellulite, at least fifteen sessions of Mesotherapy will be needed and the process should be repeated as the cellulite returns. Mesotherapy is done to avoid oral medications that have to go through the bloodstream to get to the area of the body that needs treatment. Droplets of the same medication are introduced through multiple microinjections at or around the problem spot, never too deep. Mesotherapy should be performed only by a medical doctor licensed to administer injections.

smooth operator

smooth operator

The best cure for the perfect lower half is still air brushing. Even supermodels have lumps and bumps, but you just never see them.

Nobody has smooth legs one day and dimples and lumpiness the next. The list of cellulite solutions seems endless, ranging from aromatherapy to electric muscle stimulation, and most of these techniques work only temporarily or not at all. Liposuction does not get rid of cellulite, but it does remove fatty blobs that can make your legs and lower body look thicker and rounder. A lower body lift, which is an invasive surgical procedure, can produce an overall improvement in dimpling and cellulite by lifting up the skin and tightening the muscles.

Along with banishing cellulite, select techniques that can also improve you skin tone and texture, skin elasticity, muscle tone, cell renewal, strength and stamina, and your overall body shape and posture. Any method that exfoliates the skin will improve its texture and make it feel smoother. Among these, microdermabrasion and body peels can work to wipe away dead cells from the surface. DIY methods can include loofah brush, pumice, horsehair mitts and lotions containing glycolic acid or lactic acid. Topical creams that tighten the skin can have a beneficial effect in temporarily reducing the appearance of dimpling. Of these, topical retinoids and retinol are the most effective if used on a consistent basis. Aminophylline creams may have a transient skin firming effect. To date, no topically used product can dissolve fat alone, or break up cellulite.

dos and don'ts for perfect curves

The secret is a combination of diet, exercise, and therapies. There are no quick fixes, including liposuction, which is not a cure for dimples. What you don't eat, drink, and do is more important than what you do.

- **DO** expect cellulite to become more noticeable with age as the connective tissue becomes stiffer and the skin holding the fat in place gets looser and breaks down.

- **DO** drink 6–8 glasses of water daily. Poor lymphatic flow, due to lack of physical activity and inadequate water intake, is a big contributor.

- **DO** avoid alcohol and soda. Cellulite may drive you to drink, but wine, beer and carbonated beverages will make you bloated.

- **DON'T** forget to exfoliate daily with AHA or BHA creams, and use a loofah or massage brush in the shower for stimulation and intense moisturisers to keep skin smooth.

- **DON'T** rely solely on anticellulite creams to get rid of dimpling. Most can only temporarily firm skin from the outside.

- **DON'T** waste your money on electrostimulation treatments that claim to tone your muscles but won't. Join a gym, buy a dog to run in the park with, or hire a trainer instead.

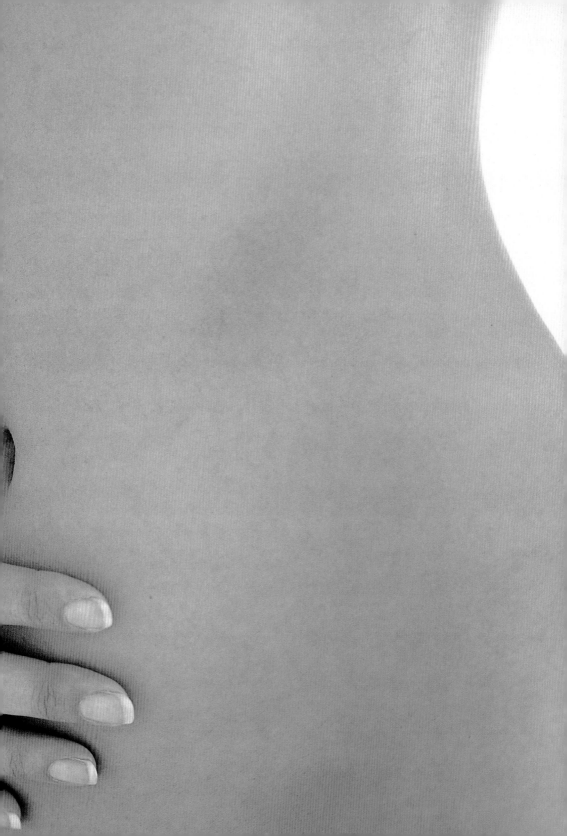

BODY CONTOURING

BODY CONTOURING

You go to the gym three times a week and watch what you eat, but you still feel like the rear end of a coach. For women striving for a better body, getting rid of unwanted fat cells sounds like a dream come true. Picture this: You go to sleep with fatty bulges and when you awake, they're gone! Liposuction is an effective way to remove unsightly bulges, giving you an improved shape and contour. This explains why liposuction, or 'lipoplasty', has long been the most popular cosmetic surgical procedure, worldwide.

Adult fat cells are incapable of multiplying. As you gain weight, they expand, and as you lose weight, they contract, but the number and distribution stay the same. This is why thin women still complain about localised fatty deposits that won't seem to budge. Liposuction reduces your overall number of fat cells and changes your shape, so any future weight gain or loss won't be as noticeable in the areas that were treated. It can jump-start a serious weight loss and exercise programme or be used as an adjunct to remove resistant bulges and improve your overall shape. In short, liposuction can be a girls' best friend.

The key to a great result from liposuction is skin quality. The tighter and firmer your skin is, the sleeker and slimmer your post-lipo shape will be. It's an operation about shape and contour.

outer limits

Liposuction is not a miracle cure – it can't give you the body of a supermodel. You can still gain weight after liposuction, but if you do, it will mostly be in areas not suctioned.

Most doctors will not perform liposuction on patients who are 2 stone or more overweight, or over 30 per cent more than their ideal body weight. If you're just 1 stone away from a size that is acceptable, lose some weight before surgery and more after. If you put on a few pounds after lipo, you'll blow your investment. If you lose some, your result will look that much better. It is not uncommon to have a small touch-up procedure 6 months later.

Liposuction works best for people who possess good skin elasticity. There are limits as to how many areas can be operated on and how much fat can be removed, based on your size, weight, and tolerance for surgery. With new techniques, amounts of 5–10 pounds of fat and fluids can be removed at one stage. If there are several areas you want suctioned, you can easily reach that level. If there is too much for one stage, the surgeon may suggest that you lose weight before having it. When skin elasticity is poor, a staged procedure is a good solution. The liposuction would be done first, and if you don't get enough skin contraction, then skin excision and internal tightening can be done at a later date, as in a tummy tuck or a thigh lift. In some cases, up to 10–20 pounds of fat may be suctioned, which is categorised as large volume lipoplasty, and is considered more risky.

Before having liposuction, your cosmetic surgeon should discuss your lifestyle, fitness level, and body-weight fluctuations. If you have a history of

YES, IT CAN

- Remove fat deposits
- Change your shape
- Take out fat from beneath the skin

NO, IT CAN'T

- Cure cellulite
- Tighten loose skin
- Take out fat from underneath muscles

an eating disorder like bulimia, anorexia or binge eating, or have been on weight-control medications, tell your surgeon in advance. Some areas of the body have fatty deposits that tend to stick around no matter how much you starve yourself or how many sit-ups you do. Fat deposits that don't respond to exercise and diet regimes are ideal spots to be liposuctioned. If you are only overweight in certain areas of your body, like the saddle bags, you would have to lose a large amount of weight in order to shrink the size of your thighs. The weight will come off from everywhere, including the breasts and face, and not just directly where you need it most. The beauty of liposuction surgery is that targets your trouble spots directly.

After liposuction there are still fat cells in the areas that were suctioned, so those body parts are not off limits. The good news is that if you do gain fat in areas of the body that weren't your primary trouble spots, it is usually very responsive to diet and exercise. For example, if you have liposuction on your stomach and you gain half a stone afterwards, it may show up on your hips. When you lose that half a stone, it will go quicker from the hips because it was the last place the fat was gained. Some women report that their breasts get fuller after having their bottom half liposuctioned, which can be an added benefit for some and unwanted side effect for others.

the art of liposuction

Liposuction has come a long way since its introduction in the mid-1970s. Modern techniques are vastly improved for women who want to make their fat cells history.

Typically, women in their twenties and thirties, go for liposuction of their inner and outer thighs and knees. In the forties and fifties, in addition to the thighs, the abdomen, hips, waist, and upper back become popular due to gaining weight with each pregnancy. By age sixty, the hips and bottom spread, and liposuction procedures give way to body lifts. As skin thins and elasticity is lost, just removing fat cells can leave sagging skin.

The procedure is very straightforward. The surgeon uses cannulas – hollow, tubular instruments with holes at one end to trap the fat. The cannula is attached to suction tubing through which the excess fat is evacuated. These instruments come in various shapes, lengths and sizes depending on the thickness and location of the fat. They have highly polished surfaces to slip through the fatty tissues with minimum friction or damage, so there is less bruising. The instruments are typically blunt-tipped to prevent cutting through the skin, and fat is suctioned out through strategically placed holes at the tip. Traditional liposuction relies on the mechanical disruption of fat cells by the movement of the cannula and the vacuum of the suction pump. Tiny incisions are made at the sites where fat is to be removed, and a wetting solution is infused to provide a numbing effect, reduce bleeding and improve fat extraction. Cannulas are inserted under the skin, moved in a back-and-forth and criss-cross fashion within the fat and then the fat is vacuumed away. The size of the cannulas used can affect the smoothness of the skin after liposuction. The use of large cannulas tends to create irregularities more often than cannulas of less than 3mm in diameter.

The output of fat is measured and the patient is checked for symmetry, although most of us have one side that is slightly fuller than the other. The procedure is completed when a safe level of fat removal is achieved. You are then monitored closely to make sure you have received enough fluid hydration and are able to urinate without difficulty. After tumescent liposuction, some blood-tinged local anaesthetic solution remains under the skin. This excess fluid is either slowly absorbed into the bloodstream or rapidly removed by draining through skin incisions. Rapid drainage reduces postoperative pain, swelling, and bruising. Surgery can be performed in hospital or at an accredited office surgery centre. For larger procedures, staying in hospital overnight may be recommended.

New studies have shown that liposuction may provide additional health benefits for some women. A dramatic reduction in body weight can be useful as a stepping-stone to long term weight loss. Large-volume liposuction (the removal of more than 10 pounds of fat) may also lead to a lowering of blood pressure and insulin levels in some women who are more than 50 pounds above their ideal weight. Strict post-op monitoring is vital after aggressive liposuction procedures.

TOP TIP:

The larger the volume of fat and fluids removed from the body, the more risky the procedure becomes and the longer the recovery is likely to be.

fat traps

Technological advances in liposuction techniques have improved results and made it safer, faster and more effective.

A major benefit of liposuction is that the scars left are tiny, less than 12mm. Small, slitlike scars can be placed in hidden areas like the belly button, the crease under the buttocks, and inside the knee. These generally heal well and are rarely visible, even in the teeniest thong.

A warmed, diluted sterile solution containing lidocaine, epinephrine, and intravenous fluid is injected into the area to be treated. As the liquid enters the fat, it becomes swollen, firm, and blanched. The expanded fat compartments allow the liposuction cannula to travel smoothly beneath the skin as the fat is removed. Saline softens the fat, adrenaline decreases the bruising, and the anaesthetic provides pain relief. For small amounts of fat, tumescent solution may be the only anaesthetic given. The solution can also be supplemented with sedatives to relax you during the procedure. General anaesthesia may be used for larger procedures involving multiple areas.

Specific risks include rare complications like pulmonary oedema – fluid in the lungs – which may occur if too much fluid is administered, and lidocaine toxicity, which can occur if there is too much lidocaine in the solution. If too much solution is injected, there is a risk of drowning in fluids. Overworking the heart is a possible consequence. There is also the possibility of a fat embolism, when a piece of fat travels into the bloodstream. Generally, the greater the volume of fat and fluids removed, the higher the chances of having a complication.

Internal ultrasound: Ultrasonic sound waves, like shock waves, are transmitted into the fatty tissues from the tip of a fine probe. Ultrasonic energy is used to liquefy or melt the fat, which is then removed using a cannula and a low-pressure vacuum. Ultrasonic liposuction is often used for large volumes and multiple areas and is good for areas where the fat is thicker and harder to get out; for example, back rolls and upper abdomen. It is usually combined with traditional liposuction when both the deeper and the more superficial fat is being removed. When previous liposuction has been done, it may be useful to soften the resulting scar tissue to make it easier for the surgeon to remove the fat.

External ultrasound: Ultrasonic energy is used in lower frequencies to soften fat deposits and smooth out bumps on the skin's surface. It is also sometimes used after liposuction to break up the hard spots and lumpiness, especially on the tummy.

Power: In 1998, the use of power was introduced to fat-sucking methods. The cannulas used are motor-driven, so they vibrate as they work, which makes removing fat easier and faster for the surgeon. The reciprocating frequency provides enough energy through the tip of the instruments to glide through fatty tissue. Since less physical exertion is required, many surgeons get better results and remove more fat. Postoperative pain, bruising, and swelling may also be reduced with this method.

Vaser: This new ultrasound technology utilises bursts of ultrasonic energy to break up fat cells for removal. Smaller, more delicate probes are used to increase the surgeon's precision and the safety of the procedure.

lipo logic

Liposuction is a very versatile procedure for women and for men. To get the best result for you, it's all about prioritising.

Starting with the face, the chin (including the neck and jowls) works well for younger people with resilient, elastic skin. Full cheeks can be minimised by liposuction as well. The upper extremities, including flabby upper arms and forearms, can be trimmed, as well as the axiliary folds (the flabby bits that peek out of a vest). Even the fatty tissues of breasts can be liposuctioned to reduce their size and heaviness. The upper and lower abdomen and waist are key areas. The upper back and back rolls that protrude around your bra and swimming costumes can be whittled down, as well as the upper hips or flanks, called 'love handles'.

The flabby folds under the bum or 'banana rolls', the outer or lateral thighs called 'saddle bags' and the inner thighs are popular areas. For heavy legs, the front and back thighs can be suctioned to reduce overall dimensions. The fleshy portion of the inner knee can be made smaller, but this area is often a combination of cartilige, bone and fat. Even heavy calves and ankles can be recontoured.

TOP TIP:
Look at your body naked in a full-length mirror. Evaluate each part separately – the upper abdomen, lower abdomen, legs, etc. To achieve the most attractive curves possible, focus on the areas you would benefit most from having recontoured. For example, if your thighs bulge, liposuctioning just one part, like the outer portion, may make the inner thighs or hips look too large in comparison.

body parts

Almost any body part can be suctioned for better contour and reduced volume, from the cheeks all the way down to the ankles.

The trend is to treat areas of the body circumferentially, instead of removing fat deposits from selected spots. Sections like the abdomen, hips, waist, and all around the thighs and knees, and upper arms, are combined to maximise the potential for skin to shrink afterwards. It is not unusual to have liposuction done in stages; for example, the lower body in one go and the trunk later.

If your greatest concern is flabby skin due to pregnancy, ageing, or yo-yo dieting, liposuction can actually make it look worse. Some fatty areas are less forgiving to major fat removal than others and more often lead to sagging skin; for example, upper arms, inner thighs, knees, abdomen, and the neck, in women over 40.

The right to bare arms

Some call them 'bat wings'; those dreaded flabby arms can really hurt someone if they swing when you wave good-bye. Along with inner thighs, upper arms are the pet hate of every woman. If you're longing to go sleeveless, intensive upper extremity exercises with weight training can help. After a certain age, when gravity has taken a toll on the thin skin of the arms, improvement won't be dramatic or quick. If you have elastic skin, liposuction can be the answer to your prayers. The upper arms can be recontoured by taking out fat through tiny incisions around the elbow. The skin contracts to a better shape after 3 weeks, when the bruising and swelling has gone. After about 3 months, you can see the final contour change. If the skin is already loose and flaccid under the arms, an arm lift (called a brachioplasty) which involves an incision made from about the elbow to the armpit, can be done. This will leave your arms slimmer and firmer, but the scar may make you feel self-conscious in a strapless top, which might defeat the purpose.

Ab flab

Women have a layer of fat stored on the abdomen. The pelvic region swells from monthly bloating, and the body adapts by outwardly stretching these muscles. Over time, the lower tummy softens and creates a bulge. Particularly in women who have had children and those in the perimenopausal range (from age 35 onwards), fat deposits tend to accumulate in the mid section of the body. If you can't remember the last time you had a waist and your hips have a mind of their own, liposuction may be able to help bring you back into belt-donning shape. The upper and lower tummy, waist, hips and flanks can be suctioned to reduce girth. It is not a substitute for a tummy tuck or abdominoplasty, but most women with reasonable firmness can get some skin shrinkage. If it is a washboard stomach you crave, a tummy tuck, which tightens the muscles and removes excess skin, is in order.

If your ultimate goal is to be taut and super trim from the waist down, a tummy tuck, thigh lift, or lower body lift are the only viable options. These involve tightening underlying muscles and removing and redraping excess skin. Unfortunately, they leave significant scarring and the recovery period is longer, but results can be amazing.

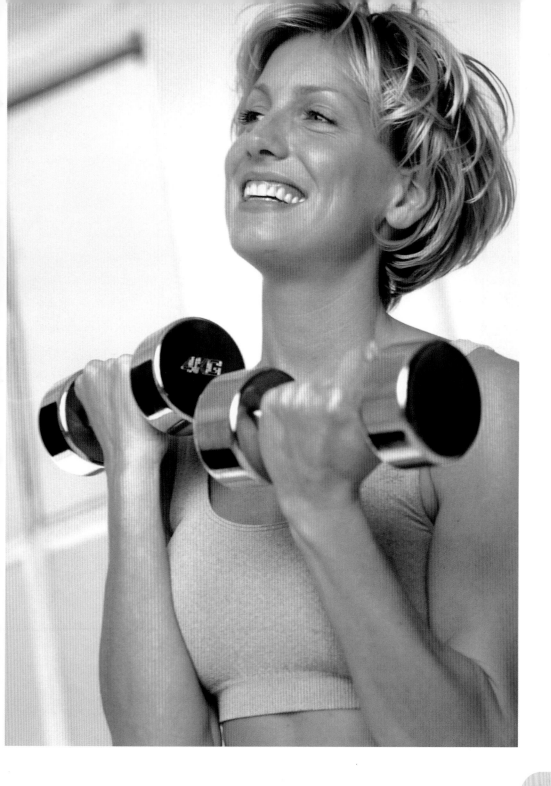

Rear views

The hips, buttocks, and thighs are undoubtedly the 'Bermuda Triangle' for women. The buttocks are the first part to lose shape due to gravity. As muscles weaken, they gradually become unable to support the fat. What one woman calls her buttocks, a cosmetic surgeon might refer to as 'lateral thighs' or 'banana rolls' – the fold of skin and fat just below the buttock crease. Another issue is how each body part flows into the next; how the buttocks are connected to the hips and outer thighs. Great rear ends have good contours and proportions; i.e. the transition from the trunk to the buttocks should be smooth and appear as though they belong to the rest of your body, instead of having a life of their own.

Improving the backside can involve taking out and putting in fat. Liposuction is rarely recommended near the buttock crease because removing the fat there can actually increase sagging. Fat from other body parts can be sucked out and injected back to smooth out your gluteus maximus, fill out dents and add curves. If you're waifish with very little body fat, a silicone buttock implant may be used to add fullness instead.

Thigh zones

The outer thighs usually respond well to liposuction and can give you a posterior view to be proud of even in your tightest-fitting jeans. The best candidates are women who are a size 10 on top and a 14 below. If you have a small backside with protruding thighs, recontouring only the buttocks may make the thighs look bigger. They are usually done as a set. The medial or inner thighs are not as thick skinned, so they

TOP TIP:
If you have had scoliosis or any type of hip injury, one side may appear higher than the other.

can sometimes look ripply or uneven after fat deposits are removed. Even the front (anterior) and back (posterior) sides of the thighs can be slimmed for a smaller overall circumference.

TOP TIP:

DON'T sit with your legs crossed with one thigh on top of the other. This impedes blood flow and can increase thigh size as waste fluids build up in the legs, causing aches, pains and cramps.

A leg up

Heavy legs are an inherited trait. If your mother or grandmother carried their weight in the thighs to the ankles, the chances are that you will too. Getting your legs fit to bare can be high maintenance. Flabby knees are the bane of any woman's existence, and all the crunches and squats on earth won't make them go away. Many women think they have Miss Piggy knees, when, in fact, it is their joints that make their knees look large and not fat at all. Liposuction can be used to delicately recontour legs from the ankles, calves and knees up to the inner and outer thighs, taking inches off the circumference of the leg. Fatty deposits can be suctioned away from the inner portion of the knees. The flabby pouches on the front of the knees are not really ideal for reduction by liposuction. Calves are often largely muscle, but suctioning even small amounts can make a big difference to the overall shape.

Liposuction of the legs takes longer than other areas to fully settle, because swelling tends to travel downward and rest below the knee. This procedure is usually best left for colder months when you can cover up bruising and swelling by wearing trousers, long skirts and opaque tights. Scars are hidden and tiny, so they won't give your secret away, and support hose will help keep swelling to a minimum. Wearing DVT stockings or support hose will help speed the swelling.

risks and recovery

Speedy healing has made the popularity of liposuction soar. You can be back at work after a long weekend. In a couple of weeks, you'll be ready for bikini season.

You can expect to have significant swelling for a few days following the procedure, but this rapidly subsides, and resolves quickly over the next few weeks. You should look good after 3 weeks and continue to improve over the next 3–6 months. Bruising is usually minimal and showering is permitted after two days. Many women return to work or some activity within 3 days for small liposuctions, 10 days for more extensive procedures. Many resume an exercise programme within 2 weeks. Postoperative pain is minimal, especially with an expertly administered anaesthetic. After 6 months, the final contour will be visible. If you are having thighs, knees or ankles done, keeping your legs elevated will reduce the swelling faster.

After surgery, a compression garment is applied to keep swelling to a minimum. Most women feel better with some compression and wear the girdle or support hose for longer. Anti-embolism boots are often used during surgery to prevent a blood clot from forming in the deep veins of the pelvis or legs. The risk of a seroma – an oozing or pooling of clear serum – is more likely in certain areas, like the abdomen, after ultrasound techniques have been used. In these cases, excess fluid may be drained to relieve pressure. Other risks apply to any surgical procedure including infection, reaction to anaesthetic, bleeding, numbness, skin loss and nerve damage. All of these are quite rare when liposuction is properly performed.

honey, I shrunk

After liposuction, most women have a better shape with fewer bulges. Clothes that were snug around the hips and thighs will flow nicely without pulling and stretching.

- You will weigh more right after liposuction than before surgery. Your face, feet and hands will swell up from all the fluids pumped into you.

- Swelling travels down like everything else, so don't be surprised if you're puffy and bruised in places you didn't have suctioned.

- Warm, aromatic baths infused with lavender and rosemary can soothe and relax sore body parts.

- Use petroleum jelly, bacitracin, or vitamin E oil to keep incisions soft and to keep scabs from forming. Don't pick at scabs, as they will take longer to heal and potentially scar.

- You may find that you itch like mad and your skin is dry and flaky. Try a rich body lotion, a loofah, and oatmeal baths.

- Avoid crash diets and appetite suppressants or diet drugs for at least two weeks after surgery. You need nourishment and lots of water, juices, and sports drinks in order to get back to optimum health.

- Don't ditch your old wardrobe or go clothes shopping for at least 6 weeks after liposuction. You will still be shrinking and won't have seen your final result yet.

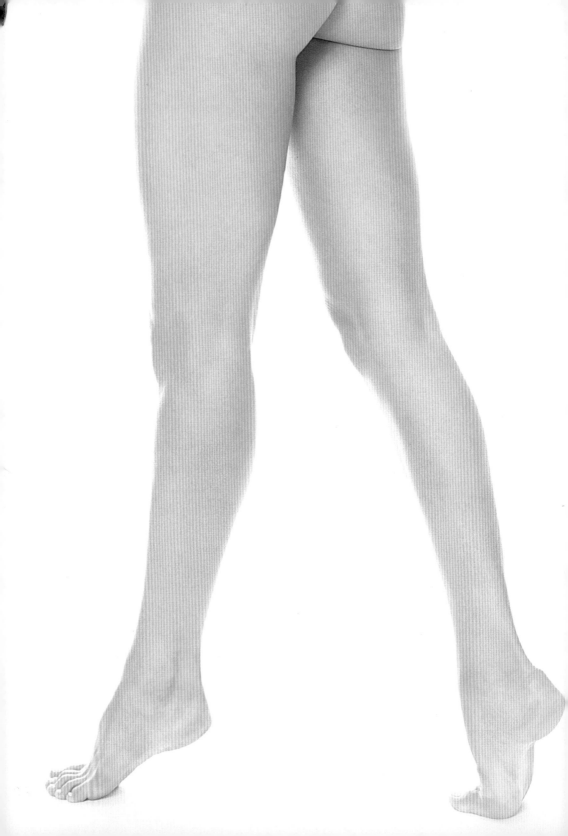

SKINNY SURGERY

SKINNY SURGERY

The last frontier in figure reshaping is the most radical. If you've done all you can at the gym and dinner table, there are still several options left to recontour your body back into beautiful form. These should be considered as the last resort, after you've done your part and lost as much weight as you can on your own.

If your skin tone is good, you are best served by liposuction. However, if you have an abundance of loose skin on the abdomen or thighs after childbirth or ageing, or have been left with a slimmer but looser body after losing a great deal of weight, liposuction won't do the job and may make your ripples look worse. When the degree of skin excess is too severe to be overcome by exercise alone, skin removal, in the form of a tummy tuck or body lift, is needed. A lower body lift is like a facelift for the body.

If you are severely obese with several dress sizes to lose to get to the size you want, gastric bypass surgery may be suggested. This procedure is undertaken to restrict your food intake so you can lose weight safely.

None of these surgical procedures are a considered quick fix, and they are not ideal for everybody. Results can be quite dramatic, but the costs, risks, potential for scarring and recovery time must factor into your decision to proceed.

obesity surgery

In the UK, nearly two-thirds of men and over half of all women are now overweight, and 1 in 5 are obese (at least 30–45 pounds overweight). The level of obesity has tripled in the past 20 years and is still raising.

Gastrointestinal surgery is a viable option for severely obese people after they have tried non-surgical approaches, or who suffer from serious obesity-related health problems. The surgery promotes weight loss by restricting food intake and interrupting the digestive process. Candidates should have a body mass index (BMI) above 40 – about 100 pounds of overweight for men and 80 pounds for women. People with a BMI between 35 and 40 who suffer from type-2 diabetes or life-threatening cardiopulmonary problems such as sleep apnea orheart disease.

The first operation widely used for severe obesity was the intestinal bypass, which produced weight loss by causing malabsorption. The concept was that if large amounts of food were eaten, they would be poorly digested or passed along too fast for the body to absorb the calories.

The Roux-en-Y: The stomach is separated and a very small pouch is created through stapling or banding to curtail food intake. A *Y*-shaped section of the small intestine is redirected to the pouch with a narrow opening, bypassing the first and second sections of the intestine to limit food absorption. The procedure requires 3 days in hospital and a 1–3 week recovery.

Restrictive surgery also serves to reduce food intake but differs from malabsorptive surgery in that it does not interfere with the digestive process.

Vertical Banded Gastroplasty: This less invasive method limits food intake by creating a small pouch in the upper stomach. The pouch fills quickly and empties slowly, producing a feeling of fullness. Overeating will result in pain or vomiting and will stretch the pouch. This procedure is performed as a day surgery and recovery takes seven to ten days.

LAP-BAND adjustable gastric banding system: A constricting ring is placed around the entire upper end of the stomach below the junction of the stomach and the oesophagus, creating an hour-glass effect, to limit food intake. No cutting or stapling is required, the outlet size is adjustable, and the band is easily removed for restoration of normal stomach anatomy. At present, there are only two devices on the market, and the Lap-Band is only freely available in the US, having been approved for use by the FDA.

These procedures can now be done laparoscopically via a fibre optic tube inserted through small incisions in the abdominal wall. Weight loss surgery is not a cure for obesity. Compulsive overeaters who don't take charge of their eating disorder can still gain weight after surgery. For more information on bariatric surgery, log on to www.asbsorg and www.naaso.org.

body lifts

If sagging and dragging are the problem, a tummy tuck or body lift may be the only answer to restore a toned, healthy body with a strong network of muscle fibres.

Tummy tuck

A tummy tuck is nearly always performed under general anesthesia in a hospital setting where you can recover overnight. There are several techniques for an abdominoplasty, the most common of which involves an incision made across the lower abdomen, just above the pubic area. This incision can be angled so it is easier to conceal. A second incision is usually made to free the navel and the surgeon tightens the underlying muscles by pulling them close together and stitching them into their new position, and extra skin is then removed. A new opening is made for the tummy button at the right position. In a mini or partial modified tummy tuck, the incision is much shorter and the navel may not need to be moved. The skin is separated only between the incision line and the navel. This skin flap is stretched down, the excess is removed and the flap is stitched back into place.

Body lift

Body lifts are the most effective technique to restore firm, youthful contours to the body. If you look in the mirror naked and pull up the saggy skin of your hips to stretch out your upper thighs and abdominal area, you can transform the way your body looks. Body lifts essentially do the same thing. The lower body lift attacks the thighs, buttocks, abdomen, waist, and hips all in one stage. The added benefits are an overall improvement in dimpling and cellulite, as well as the elevation of a woman's private parts to a more youthful status. It requires an incision around the entire circumference of the abdominal area to remove flabby skin and lift the flank, thigh, and buttocks areas. The incision can usually be placed discreetly within standard or high-cut bikini lines.

The fat is lifted off the muscle and the hanging skin is elevated and tacked into a higher position. Stitches are placed in layers to the deeper structures below and attached to hold the fat and skin securely in place. The scars are extensive and recovery is longer than most other cosmetic surgical procedures, about 3 weeks. Often, multiple stages are required if there are many areas of hanging skin; for example, the lower torso, breasts and arms, and inner thighs and knees. If inner thighs and saggy knees are the problem, a medial or inner thigh lift is required. For this a horizontal incision is generally placed in the groin area and excess skin is lifted and removed. These scars can often drop over time as the skin loosens up.

Expert advice

For any surgery involving wide incisions, smokers should be very cautious, as nicotine interferes with wound healing and can increase the risks of infection and poor scars.

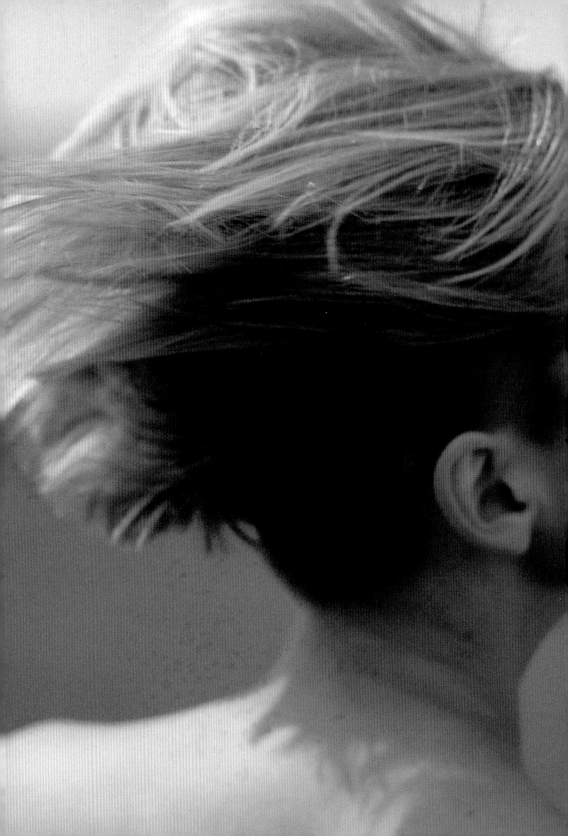

HAIR AFFAIR

HAIR AFFAIR

Never underestimate the power of great hair. It is the frame around your face, the finishing touch to your total look. It is an essential part of your image and can be a beautiful accessory.

It's one of the first things you notice about a woman, right up there with eyes and lips.

A great style is the ultimate fashion statement. Hairstyles change every season, but whatever the look, thick is always in. Both women and men tend to be most attracted to a head of hair that is dense, long, and a good colour. The goal is shine, softness, strength, and 'stylability', which are key indicators of healthy hair and what every woman craves.

The expression 'bad hair day' has become a part of our vernacular. Its closest translation: If your hair doesn't look good, you don't look good. Thin, limp, or stringy hair makes you feel like a 'plain Jane'. An updated style is the quickest path to reinventing yourself. Faking it can be the next best thing. Today, there are quick, effective methods to give you the mane you wish you were born with. The other important hair cares for women are hair removal and controlling facial hair growth and unruly brows. Unfortunately, we never seem to have enough hair where we want it and we have too much where we don't.

clean regime

Just like your face, your hair needs a cleansing ritual for the morning, the evening and emergencies. These may change with the seasons.

Great-looking hair starts in the shower. Go gently on your follicles to maintain each strand for as long as you can and to keep them bouncy. Over-cleansing, pulling and tugging, and too much styling and fixing can weaken hair and make it brittle. Many shampoo bottles have directions that instruct you to shampoo and rinse twice. The idea is that the first removes dirt, oil, and product build-up and the second helps add volume, as well as providing a backup in case the first shampoo didn't get your hair clean enough. However, for dry or brittle hair, one shampoo may be enough.

The presence of airborne pollutants and holes in the ozone layer, and the use of steam heat, hot rollers, and blow-dryers means your hair tends to attract dust and dirt. For some women, daily washing with a shampoo formulated to restore balance to the hair and scalp is a necessity. Others are happy to skip a day or two. For short hair, daily washing is usually needed. Every other day for longer hair may be suitable, especially since the time involved to dry and style can be more than you can manage. Washing hair more than once a day is not necessary. The natural oils produced each day provide thickness and shine that you don't want to strip away by over-washing. There are some women who can get away with seeing their stylist once a week for a wash and blow dry, but that is rare.

shampoo selection

Selecting the right products for your hair type and condition will help you make the most of it. Start with the basics and add as needed. Your hair may grow tired of a product before you do.

Shampoos for coloured, permed, or processed hair: Chemically processed hair needs special formulas that won't strip colour and contain ingredients that are gentle and moisturizing.

Highlighting or colour-enhancing shampoos: Designed to prevent colour from fading, they add tone and extend the life of your highlights. They add shine to grey hair and help reduce yellow. They are also good to use after a permanent, as the peroxide in neutralizers can lighten the colour of your hair.

Clarifying shampoos: These contain an acidic ingredient, such as apple cider, lemon juice or vinegar, to cut through residue built up by styling products. Use these before you colour, perm or relax your hair to allow the treatment to be absorbed better and go on more evenly. They are too drying to use every day; once or twice a week is enough. Overuse can cause excess stripping of the natural oils.

Volumizing or body-building shampoo: These contain proteins that bond to the hair to add volume. Use them sparingly, as overuse may build up residue. For fine hair, alternate with a regular shampoo. Look for ingredients like 'dimethicone copolyol'; a silicon derivative that helps to build volume in hair.

conditioner choices

Conditioners make the hair smoother and add body and shine, but there is a fine line between the right amount of conditioner and too much.

Conditioners are usually made of large molecules that literally stick to the outside of the hair and make combing easier, which prevents the hair from twisting and breaking. Hair tangles when the cuticle doesn't lie flat and the hairs can't slide past one another with ease. Because they coat the hair, conditioners make it look shiny and protect it from damage from the environment and styling tools. They usually contain silicone and moisture-producing substances like ceramides and complex lipids that smooth over hair and can reduce frizz and static electricity.

Although conditioners can add thickness and volume to thin or thinning hair, over-conditioning may cause it to look greasy. It can cause the cuticle layer to lift, making it brittle. Whether you use conditioner or not depends on your hair. For thin hair, use only lightweight, rinse-out conditioners. Volumisers with ingredients like keratin, collagen, and hydrolyzed proteins help to plump up strands for fuller-looking hair. Chemically processed hair needs conditioner to counteract the drying and damaging effects of the dyes and peroxides.

TOP TIP:
Conditioners should be at a low pH of 4.0–4.5 to maintain the protein in the hair.

Most of us don't give conditioners time to work. Don't rinse before the conditioner has had a chance to seep into the hair. Wait at least 5 minutes.

Dry hair
Leave-in conditioners

These treatments are usually applied to towel-dried hair. They coat the hair, making it heavier and weighing it down. Some formulas have UV protection built in to protect hair from sun, wind, and heat.

Dry and damaged hair
Deep conditioners

They include proteins and moisturising ingredients to repair split ends and brittleness. They are usually left on for 10–30 minutes and rinsed out thoroughly.

Hot oils

Massage a few drops directly into the scalp every 2–4 weeks. Apply lightly to avoid overgreasing.

Fine and curly hair
Thickening serums

Proteins and polymers are bound to the hair shaft, making hair fuller. Apply to wet hair before styling.

Detanglers

These work well as a substitute for conditioner on both fine and curly hair. Choose a light formula and rinse out thoroughly before combing hair.

Most hair types
Rinse-out conditioners

These increase shine, smooth the hair cuticle, soften the hair, and reduce static. They are used after shampooing and should be rinsed out thoroughly.

*All-in-one shampoo-
and-conditioners*

Shampoo/conditioner combos leave a residue that builds up quickly and weighs hair down. They should never be used on oily hair. Best reserved for travel.

the white stuff

The condition of your scalp can provide a clue to the health of your hair. A healthy scalp provides a strong foundation for a gorgeous, shiny head of hair.

Part your hair in a place near the crown where you can see it in the mirror. Run a fine-tooth comb gently across the scalp. See how much flaking you pick up. Some occasional flaking is normal and doesn't necessarily mean you have dandruff. It could be a form of dermatitis or eczema. Dandruff is characterized by a dry, itchy scalp and white flakes that show up on your shoulders, especially when you're wearing dark colours. Dandruff is a normal shedding of skin, and is actually a form of seborrhea that is more common in men than in women. The exact cause is unknown but contributing factors can include stress, sweating and hormones.

Dandruff can be present in dry or oily scalps, but is more common in oily skin types. The key to controlling dandruff is to remove the flakes as soon as they appear by frequent washing with a medicated shampoo, which not only removes the dandruff but also cuts down on the rate of shedding. For most sufferers, dandruff is a lifetime condition that can be controlled by using the right shampoo.

TOP TIP:
African and black women tend to have drier hair, which is likely to attract flakes. Daily shampooing may not be necessary. Massage the scalp to stimulate your natural oils. A light-textured oil can be used on the scalp, or ask your doctor about using a shampoo that contains a steroid.

Over-the-counter medicated shampoos usually contain coal tar, salicylic acid (beta hydroxy acid), selenium sulphide, or zinc pyrithione. Prescription strength sulphur, ketoconazole, and topical steroids may also be used. If your hair is processed, avoid products with selenium sulphide or sulphur.

Severe forms of dandruff, where flakes are oilier and more yellowish than usual and the scalp is red and inflamed, might be Seborrheic Dermatitis, which requires treatment from a doctor. Use every day until your dandruff disappears. For maintenance, use medicated shampoos only as needed to avoid drying out your hair. Use a shampoo and conditioner for dry hair the rest of the time.

- **DON'T** use heavy conditioners and styling products designed to coat the hair, as they can prevent the natural shedding of the scalp. This may cause a build-up of flakes.

- **DO** switch to a gentler product, which may reduce flaking if your scalp is reacting to a harsh ingredient in your shampoo.

- **DO** use a clarifying shampoo that contains cider, which may reduce product buildup and help to clear the scalp of flakes.

- **DO** use tea tree oil, which can be helpful as an antiseptic.

- **DO** give yourself regular scalp massages.

- **DO** try to avoid centrally heated rooms as dry scalp conditions can be aggravated by a lack of moisture in the air.

oil spills

Hair has natural oils secreted from the sebaceous glands to protect hair and keep it shiny. Oily hair may be greasy at the scalp, but dull and dry at the ends.

Fine, thin hair is the most prone to looking oily and limp. Wash hair daily with a mild shampoo that does not contain a conditioner so it leaves the least amount of residue. Formulas specifically for oily hair and clarifying shampoos work well. Use only a very light conditioner or a diluted formula on the ends only and rinse out thoroughly.

Greasy hair needs conditioning, too, just less of it. Avoid products containing silicone, mineral oils, and lanolin, which coat the hair, weigh it down, and make the strands lie flat against the scalp. If your hair has become stringy by midday, spritz water on it and comb through to remove and redistribute oils. The goal is to avoid stripping away all the natural oils.

In humid weather, you may shower and wash your hair more often, especially if it is oily. Switch to a gentle shampoo for frequent use. If you sweat a lot when exercising, shampoo after your workout.

It is time to switch shampoos if:

- You like your hair better the morning after you've washed it.
- Your hair feels weighed down and you feel the need to rinse it more.
- Your hair is hard to detangle or style.
- Your hair doesn't look shiny.
- Sudsing no longer gives you a rich lather.

On rainy days, hair attracts moisture, which can make it go wild and very elastic. Fix it with a finishing spray to keep it where you want it.

Oil overdrive

Excess oil means your sebaceous glands are in overdrive. The waxy oil these glands produce not only gives hair a greasy appearance but also builds up on the scalp. When sebum hardens, it blocks blood flow and starves the roots embedded in the scalp. The roots are weakened and hair loss can occur. Excess oil makes your head a magnet for dirt, sometimes giving it the appearance of a string mop.

Scalp check-up: Part your hair at the crown and blot your scalp with a soft white tissue. If any residue shows, you have an oily scalp.

Magic hands

Nothing beats massage to stimulate blood flow to the scalp, keep your hair in peak condition and relax you from head to toe. Massage has not been scientifically proven to stimulate new hair growth. Begin by wetting your hair. Choose one of the natural ingredients listed below, depending on the condition of your scalp. Add a splash to some warm mineral water to make a solution. Drizzle the mixture through your hair, massaging as you go.

Dry or tight scalp: Warm almond oil, sesame oil, or a light olive oil.
Greasy scalp: Astringents like witch hazel, lemon juice, and cider vinegar.
Normal scalp: Softening ingredients like jojoba and aloe.

mane class

When it comes to hair care, think seasonally. During the winter, there's no humidity in the air, so hair flattens out as it loses moisture. Switch to lighter products and nongreasy formulas. For summer's high humidity, go with formulas that slick hair down and maintain shape and shine.

Problem: Frizzy

For curly hair, work anti-frizz gel through hair and blow-dry using a diffuser attachment. For straight hair, apply straightening cream, then divide hair into sections. Using a big round brush to hold hair taut, blow-dry each section, aiming air down the hair shaft. Finish with a straightening iron after hair is dry.

Fast fix: Finger-dry roots to avoid overheating. Use a lightweight detangling spray. Rub finishing emulsion between your palms and smooth over any frizz.

Problem: Greasy

For oily hair that needs frequent washing, avoid using shine-enhancing products, which can make greasy hair look stringy. Don't use creamy conditioners and waxes that stay on the hair shaft and put your oil production into overdrive. Don't over-brush. Use a dab of leave-in conditioner on the ends only, avoiding the scalp.

Fast fix: Blot your scalp with oil-absorbing sheets intended for your face.

Problem: Lanky or limp

Shampoo with a volumizing product, then apply a light conditioner to the ends. When your hair is 60 per cent dry, apply 5–10 spritzes of body-boosting spray to your roots. While blow-drying, lift sections of your hair with fingers or a vent brush and aim heat at the roots.

Fast fix: Lift your hair at the roots and spritz with light, flexible-hold spray.

Problem: Fly-away

Static electricity is caused by friction between your comb and your hair, and between individual hairs. Don't comb too often. Conditioners coat the hair, which provides insulation. Use the highest-level conditioner you can that doesn't weigh your hair down.

Fast fix: Lightly spray on leave-in conditioner or apply drops of silicone serum.

Problem: Porous

Porous hair will quickly soak up whatever you put on it, as well as the humidity in the air. If your hair gets frizzy on muggy days and flat on very dry ones, it's probably porous. Coarse, permed, straightened or processed hair is often porous, as well as hair that has been damaged.

Fast fix: Use a rich conditioner and leave on as long as possible. Look for products containing proteins and humectants, especially at the ends. Silicone serums can help smooth down the cuticle and add shine.

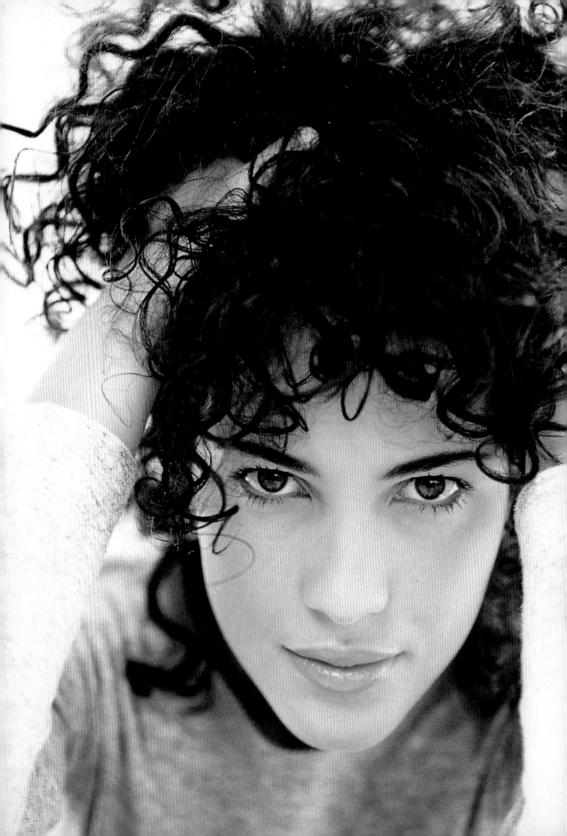

MANAGING IT

MANAGING IT

Half the battle is learning how to work with the head of hair you've got. You may know how your hair behaves and what pitfalls to avoid, but getting hair to look healthy, shiny, and manageable can take a lot of practice and first-hand expert advice.

The best cuts are easy to style on your own and versatile so you can get a lot of looks from them. It all starts at the salon. It is hard to take a step back and figure out your hair options for yourself. A good stylist can look at you objectively and know what will work for you and what won't.

Every woman can have a bad hair day once in a while. There are days when you just can't be bothered or don't have the extra time it takes to devote to your style. Make a contingency plan. Your stylist can teach you the tricks you need to throw together a great look. Learning how to tie hair back, pile it up or twist it around can be a lifesaver when you're pressed for time. Arm yourself with the best tools for your hair and have your own stylist teach you how to use them in emergencies. For example, the perfect hairdryer with the correct brush size and bristle, and the optimum performance straightening iron. For special occasions, a quick blow-dry by a professional is well worth the expense. No one can make your hair look as gorgeous and glam as an extra pair of talented hands.

scissor hands

scissor hands

Keep hair in peak condition with frequent trims. Whether long or short, hair should be trimmed on a regular basis, every 6–8 weeks.

Waiting too long between cuts allows ends to become susceptible to breakage. There is no miracle product to repair split ends. The only way to get rid of them is to cut them off. Short of a great haircut, the best split-end treatment is a leave-in conditioner with light hold or a pomade applied to the ends to temporarily seal the splits. When growing out layers, make sure you have a reshape on a regular basis to keep hair healthy and maintain maximum fullness.

TOP TIP:
Don't skimp. One of the best beauty investments you can make is to get a great hairdresser.

Stylists are usually the first people to notice problems such as hair loss. They have the advantage of being able to see the back of your head. Find a hairdresser you bond with and who will be honest if there is a problem.

If you are trying to grow out layers or a fringe, you need frequent visits to the salon to maintain a style. Unless you're desperate, don't trim your hair yourself. Most professional stylists will allow you to pop in to have your fringe trimmed inbetween haircuts to keep your style in check.

To do it yourself, follow these tips to get the job done right. Use a straight comb with wide teeth, very sharp haircutting scissors (not the ones in your kitchen drawer), and gel to give you added control. Secure the rest of your hair, leaving only the fringe hanging loose to avoid any accidents. A soft, wispy fringe that sweeps along the eyebrows is the most flattering and should frame your upper face and brow area. The endpoint is your brow bone. A short, choppy fringe or cut straight across can look more severe.

Many women over 40 enjoy the benefits of covering up forehead lines, wrinkles, and creases. A well-tailored fringe can camouflage an ageing forehead or hairline that is too high. It can also save you a fortune in Botox shots.

Stop tearing your hair out

Ponytails and tight plaits tug on hair and cause breakage. Use covered hair bands rather than the rubber ones you'll find in your desk drawer. Scrunchies, cloth-covered bands and ribbons are a good alternative to thin elastic bands. The wider the band, the less tension on the hair. Vary where you place your ponytails from day to day, especially those placed high on the head, and give your hair a day off regularly to limit the stress on your hair. Be especially careful when you remove bands, clips and barrettes from your hair because you can pull out hair that gets tangled in them. Choose clips that do not have sharp edges. Bungee elastics that have a hook at each end can be used to pull hair into a ponytail or bun without making knots, by wrapping them around your hair until it is tight enough and then hooking the ends together.

the search for a stylist

Finding the right stylist is like dating – it's a long-term relationship and chemistry counts. Communication is also key. It may take time to get to know and understand each other.

- Ask for recommendations from friends and other beauty professionals. If you see a woman with a hairstyle that you really like, ask her who she goes to.

- Go for a complementary consultation. Look around at the stylists and clients. Don't just put your head into someone's hands on a first visit.

- Get a list of prices for all the treatments offered to avoid a shock later. Choose a stylist you can afford to encourage more frequent visits.

- Tell your stylist about your lifestyle, what you do for a living, and how much time you have to devote to your hair.

- Communicate the type of look and length you're going for and if you wear glasses, take them with you.

- If you don't like the way the cut is turning out, stop the stylist immediately to discuss it.

- If you think a different stylist in the same salon might suit you better, you can switch, even though it may feel awkward.

- One bad haircut doesn't mean you should switch stylists if you have been happy in the past. Talk it over with the stylist.

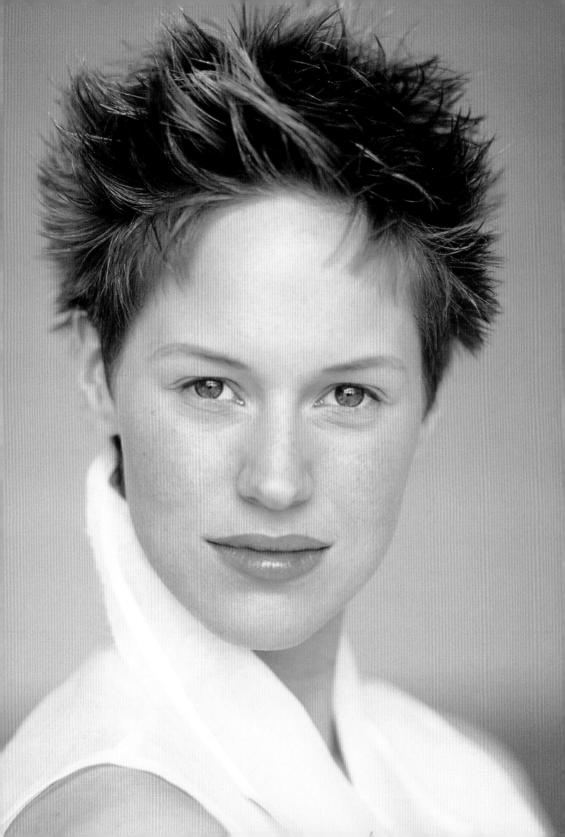

hot stuff

Of the many styling tools that use heat, the blow-dryer is the most commonly used. Curling irons come in second.

Nothing achieves a fuller look than a blow-dryer in well-trained hands – it is an indispensable tool. However, the heat produced by styling tools can make chemical changes in hair, which can have a negative effect on surface lipids and protein structure. Heat can literally boil out the water content in the hair shaft as it turns to steam, which damages the cortex. Over-exposure to heat will make any type of hair look and feel lifeless.

The heat is on

Approach heat tools with caution, especially if your hair is not in good condition. Always hold a blow-dryer at least 6 inches from your scalp and vary the temperature settings, using high heat only for short spurts. Keep it moving; don't hold it on one spot for too long. The hair concentration nozzle helps keep hot coils as far away from the scalp as possible. A narrow plastic nozzle with a thin slit directs heat on one area at a time without ruining the adjacent section that you finished drying. To dry like a pro, divide and conquer. Section off the front into thirds and secure each part with a clip. For thicker hair, make more sections. Diffusers – the cone-shaped attachments that fit on the barrels of blow-dryers – are good for diffusing the

BEAUTY BYTE:

For more tips on hair care, try
www.behindthechair.com.

airflow over a larger area and drying hair more slowly. These work well for curly hair to hold the curl. The most effective blow-dryer should have enough power to get the job done – from 1,200–2,000 watts. Beware of cheaper models that often use more heat than needed.

The same rules apply to curling irons. Go for one with a cool tip designed to use easily with one hand. Some models have an automatic safety shut-off switch to control the temperature settings. You can bake a cake at about 180°C, so imagine what your curling tongs are doing to your hair with their average temperature of 140°C. Blow-dryers are slightly cooler at 120°C, while hot rollers usually work at 100°C.

Ceramic pressing irons are the next best thing to professional straightening. Better models can achieve higher temperatures than conventional models which cuts your styling time in half. For bleached or fragile hair, the lower setting is advised. For coarse or thick hair, maximum heat on a high setting works best. Use an iron after hair has been blown dry.

If you've been on an all-out blow-drying mission lately, your hair may feel like damaged goods. Give it a rest and time to repair itself. Try an absorbent hair towel that can dry hair in record time. Towel drying can rough up the cuticle, which makes hair harder to comb through. Squeeze out excess water and wrap hair in a towel. Air-dry your hair naturally to avoid damage for a change.

Some conditioning and styling products are heat-activated to get treatment directly where the potential for damage is greatest. They can slow down keratin breakage and stimulate the metabolism of the hair root.

frazzled follicles

frazzled follicles

Dry hair is a relative concept. Hair can react dramatically to the way you treat it. You may think your hair is dry because of insufficient moisture and oil content.

If your hair does not have a normal sheen or texture but is dry and brittle, it may be the result of excessive washing, harsh detergents, heat processing, or a dry or hostile environment. Friction is another culprit. Rough brushing or over-combing, even fabric pillows and pillowcases, can cause friction on the hair, which can be potentially damaging.

One way to combat the coarse, brittle texture of dry hair is by using conditioners. If your hair is on the dry side, use a conditioner after every shampoo to achieve softness and shine. Even conditioners cannot revitalize severely damaged hair. If your hair is constantly dry and intensive conditioning doesn't seem to help, see your doctor. Fragile hair that breaks easily may be a sign of more than just a problem of vanity. It may be caused by an underlying medical condition, such as metabolic diseases, hypothyroidism, or poor nutrition.

Abnormally dry, lifeless hair may also be a result of the natural oil being stripped from the cuticle due to any of a number of causes. Hair tends to dry out during the winter in cold climates and can become dry after the use of steam heat, long periods of sun exposure, or when there us a build-up of flakes, clogs and oil glands. Over processing with chemicals and heat are the worst culprits – and the easiest to avoid.

damage control

damage control

Damaged hair needs extra tender loving care. The first step should always be prevention. Once the damage is done, it is harder to get from dull back to diva.

- **DO** apply a drop of shine-enhancing serum or cream to damp hair after washing.

- **DO** use a shine-enhancing spray if you have straight hair. Mist all over. Straight hair is prone to flattening fast.

- **DO** allow your hair to dry naturally whenever possible, or dry just the top layer with a blow-dryer to avoid heat damage.

- **DO** use a conditioner or a few drops of olive oil on the ends of your hair twice a week. Cover hair with a towel and leave on for 20 minutes.

- **DO** use a humidifier in your home to replace any moisture loss, especially in cold weather when home heating is used. Curly hair tends to need more added moisture. For emergency repair, try a deep conditioning masque overnight.

lifestyle lessons

The environment can wreak havoc with your hair. Exposure to UV rays has the same effect on your hair as it has on your skin.

Environmental damage causes physical changes in your hair, including the destruction of cuticle cells, roughening of the hair surface, loss of elastic strength, and increased porosity, or the ability to absorb moisture. Damage shows up more easily in lighter hair colours.

Hair enemies

The enemy	Hair protection
Saltwater	Rinse or wash your hair after swimming in the sea.
Sun exposure	Wear a hat or scarf; use a spray with a sunscreen.
Steam heat	Use a humidifier at night; apply a conditioning treatment weekly.
Chlorinated pools	Wash hair immediately after swimming.
Extreme temperatures	Wear a hat to keep hair covered.
Wind	Keep hair pulled back; wear a cap.
Pollution	Use a spray with a sunscreen; use clarifying products.

Any harsh natural condition can have a negative impact on the quality and strength of your hair. When hair is damaged, dirt and other particles can get lodged between the scales, making hair look dull. Grey hair is particularly susceptible to damage from the sun, which can give it a yellowish tint. Sunscreens have been created especially for hair that contain protection that filters out UV rays. They can be found in leave-in conditioners, detanglers, and finishing sprays. They are most effective in products that are not rinsed out, and can be re-applied during the day as needed, or after swimming. If your hair is exposed to the sun a lot, avoid using a blow-dryer. Sun and blow-drying present the worst possible combination for your hair.

Working hair

A day at the office can cause stress on your strands. The lack of moisture in recycled office air can strip hair and leave it looking dull and flat. Frizziness and static is not far behind. Heat from heating systems, fluorescent lighting and overhead bulbs contribute to dryness. When your work environment is warm or humid, you start to sweat. Sweat contains salt, which gets lodged in your hair and can cause dehydration. Perspiration from anxiety and running around can also be hard on the hair and flatten out your style before lunchtime. As the day progresses, your hair may need a pick-me-up. Cany emergency supplies – a mini pressing iron – can be a quick way to cut down on frizz.

BEAUTY BYTE:

For more information on high-tech hair care ingredients, visit www.uspto.gov/patft

mold it

Styling products can add shine and texture, as well as control flyaway hairs. The goal is to set your style once and maintain it for as long as possible throughout the day.

The worst mistake that women make is to use too many products that have conflicting or overlapping missions at the same time. Determine your hair type and stick with just enough to get the style you want and keep it, but no more. Each product will leave some ingredients on the hair that can weigh it down. Typically, a little bit goes a long way no matter what type of hair you have. Hair should always be soft, silky, and irresistibly touchable.

Less is definitely more; the thicker or stickier the styling product, the less you need. The less you touch or handle your hair, the better it looks. The finer or thinner your hair, the less product you should use. Overcompensating via extra styling can lead to hair disaster – learn when to leave well enough alone.

Gels and mousses: Designed to hold, add shine and texture, gels come in lighter, user-friendly spray-on formulas for even distribution. They are generally worked through the entire head to give hair some shape, form, and staying power. A light gel can help add body and volume to your hair, but thick, gloopy gels weigh hair down. For fine, thinning hair, look for gels that offer thickening, and light or medium hold. Mousses are light and foamy and work well for finer, curly hair, but tend to be more drying.
Directions: Use on clean hair that is partially dry or damp, rather than on dripping wet hair when they weigh strands down. Avoid applying before

using curling tongs, since the heat may cause your hair to stick to the tongs if the gel or mousse melts down. Use a small dollop (the size of a one-pound-coin) squeezed into your palm, rub palms together to spread evenly and apply lightly. Use fingertips to scrunch waves and curls, and an open palm to create a smoother, sleeker look. For longer hair, applying fixatives from midway down the hair will give a better hold. Comb through if needed to distribute evenly. Applying gels near the roots or brushing products through the hair will flatten out your curls.

Sprays: Styling sprays create a style, whereas holding sprays keep it in place. Stiff hairsprays are a no-no. Avoid products labelled 'maximum hold', which defeat the purpose of adding volume by making hair sticky. Sprays containing alcohol tend to be more drying; ditto for aerosols. Non-aerosols often provide less hold, but give a more natural look and feel. If your hair is thin or limp, use a fine misting spray. Holding sprays may contain polymers that act as a fixative. The finer the mist, the smaller the droplets deposited. Sprays also keep humidity out, which keeps your style in shape.
Directions: Spray a small amount evenly over your style from a distance of about 30cm. Don't spritz too close to the hair, as this will cause build-up. You may reapply later in the day, so don't overuse.

Waxes and pomades: Reserved for thick, curly and coarse hair types and should never be used on fine or limp hair. Waxes are heavier than pomades and create spiky styles or tame unruly ends. Pomades are applied to slick hair down and keep it frizz-free in humid weather.
Directions: Use only a dab rubbed on the palms and/or fingertips, distribute evenly through the hair. Use sparingly to avoid a greasy, flat look.

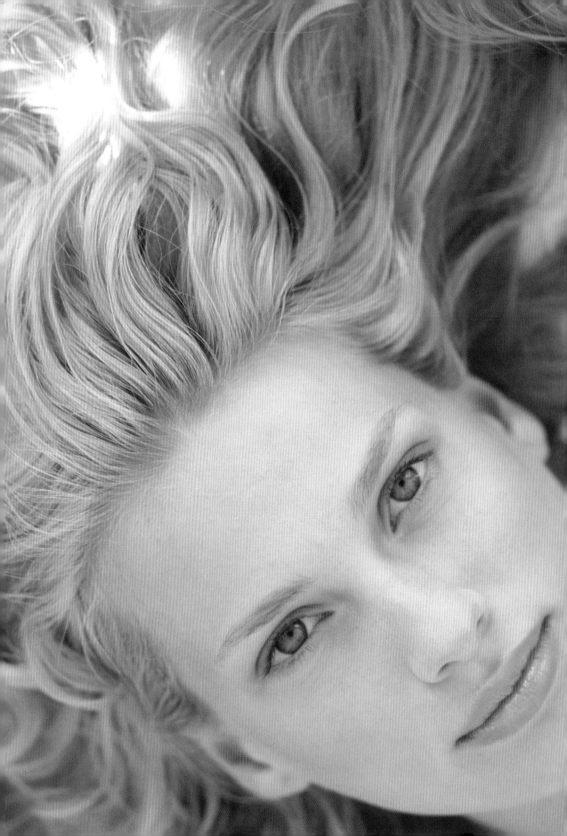

PROCESSING IT

PROCESSING IT

Technology has made great progress in hair processing, so you no longer have to be stuck with the head of hair you were born with. At one time, covering grey represented the major market in hair dyes. Today, women no longer wait until they see their first grey hair to enhance their natural colour.

Instead of damaging follicles, colour is beneficial to hair and the best method of adding volume and lift. The colouring process plumps up the hair cuticle, fattens each strand, and adds texture and shine.

Your natural hair colour is determined by the type of melanin present. Eumelanins produce black or brown hair. Pheomelanins produce blondes or redheads. The colour, and I mean your 'natural' colour, also says something about the amount and type of hair. The more pigment in your hair, the darker its colour. As we age, pigment fades and the hair turns grey. When pigment is lost altogether, the hair becomes white. As if we didn't know already, blondes – with around 120,000 hairs compared to brunettes with an average of 100,000 hairs – not only have more fun, they also have more hair.

New methods for hair straightening have revolutionized the process, making glorious, silky tresses possible for naturally unmanageable hair. A professional thermal reconditioning treatment can last 4-6 months. Many women swear that it's the best thing they have ever done for their locks.

relaxed attitude

Going from curly to straight or stick straight to corkscrews can be an uphill battle. If you do fancy a change, try a less dramatic one first like straight or curly to soft waves.

Chemical relaxers applied to frizzy or kinky hair can be very damaging to your follicles and may also lighten hair slightly. Thermal reconditioning is a method of permanently straightening or relaxing over-curly hair. Unlike previous hair straightening methods, these systems can be done on most hair types except hair that has been over processed and highlighted, where the risk of damage goes up exponentially. Ammonium thioglycolate is the main solution used which has a lower pH balance than more caustic agents in regular straightening products. Better quality products have a lower percentage of active ingredient and lower pH balance of ammonium thioglycolate. The best thermal irons can reach temperatures of up to 356°F. The heat and method of pressing the hair with a special iron that helps restructure the hair bonds so that it lies straight, and requires barely any blow-drying. It improves the texture, softness and shine, and makes hair very manageable. The ironing process takes considerable skill, patience and practice, and may take 4–8 hours. Repeat treatments will be required in 4–6 months for

FOLLICLE FACT:

Curl varies according to ethnicity.

- Asian, Indian – the cortex is round, so the hair tends to be straight.
- African, Black – the cortex is flattened and curved, so the hair is more curly.
- White, Caucasian – slender, cylindrical with varying curves, so the hair can range from straight to curly.

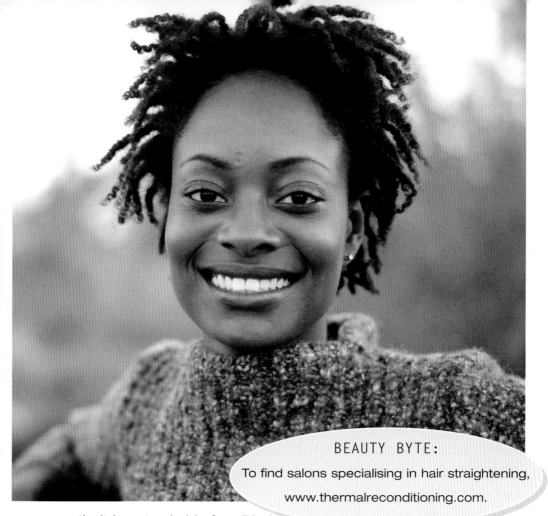

BEAUTY BYTE:

To find salons specialising in hair straightening,

www.thermalreconditioning.com.

new growth. It is not suitable for all hair
types and pin straight hair is not flattering to all faces.

Go curl

The safest way to add curls is to use regular rollers and wind hair loosely around them. Heated rollers can be used safely if they have fabric coverings to protect hair from breakage. Velcro rollers are a universal favourite. Use them on dry hair for 20 minutes to reduce frizz and add body and control. Hot sticks, mouldable foam or plastic tubes are gentle on hair, but the look is more tousled than precision curls.

the right shade

the right shade

Colouring your own hair is not for the weak at heart. Getting it right may look easy but it isn't foolproof.

Dye can leave a mess in your sink and stains on your towels and on your hands if you don't use gloves. The safest place to start is with a semi-permanent colour and follow the directions religiously. Always do a strand test to get the timing right. Many formulas are developed to stop working once the required time has elapsed to prevent disasters. If you have a particularly sensitive scalp, do a patch test the first time to make sure you don't end up with a rash or irritation. Cream formulas are more buffered than liquids, and the lower the pH, the gentler on your follicles.

TOP TIP: Applying a moisturiser around your hairline and ears will help prevent the colour from staining your skin.

Bathroom blondes tend to look like they did it themselves. If the shade you choose isn't quite right, you'll need an expensive salon visit to sort things out. Have a professional do your colour the first time. Strategically lightening selected strands of hair can give the most natural look. Tints can also be used that lift and deposit colour in only one step. If your base colour is very dark, a rinse can be used before highlights to reduce the contrast. Highlighting livens up flat, dull, monocoloured hair and adds texture and variations of shades throughout. If you want to mimic the effects of a day at the beach, use the lightest shade at the top of your head. Subtle highlights add brightness and warmth that can enhance your skin tone.

Permanent colour: The most popular hair dye, but the most damaging. Two chemicals make permanent colours work: hydrogen peroxide (the developer or activator) and ammonia. These swell the cuticle, remove natural pigment and deposit dye. This process damages the hair cuticle and destroys protein. For your first time, go to a professional who can custom-mix colours and minimise damage.

Lasts: 4–6 weeks (after which time roots will need retouching)

Semi-permanent colour: Gentler than permanent dyes, these liquid, gel, or foam formulas penetrate the hair shaft and stain the cuticle without peroxide or ammonia. The colour fades with every shampoo, meaning roots aren't as noticeable. If your hair is already damaged from perming or straightening, this is the gentlest process possible.

Lasts: 6–8 weeks

Temporary colour: Includes colour-enhancing shampoos and conditioners, as well as rinses and toners that deposit a translucent layer of dye on the outside of the cuticle. They are a good way to create highlights, camouflage small amounts of grey or freshen permanent or semi- permanent colours.

Lasts: 4–6 shampoos

BEAUTY BYTE:

To go it alone, log on to
www.haircolorwizard.com before you dye.

true colours

true colours

Just like the skin, your hair is subject to damage from handling and external influences. Any treatment or process has the potential to break hair.

Both the hair and scalp can be traumatised by perming and straightening chemicals. Bleached and dyed hair can be weakened if chemicals are used too often, or if the solution is left on the hair too long. They key culprits are peroxide and ammonia.

Once your hair has been chemically altered, the risk of damage from regular use of heated styling tools goes up exponentially. Permed or straightened hair is more porous than normal hair, so it absorbs dyes more quickly. Abusing colour-treated hair can make it feel like straw. Sun oxidizes and fades your colour – so cover your head when in intense sunlight.

Green team

To avoid turning your gorgeous colour a vivid shade of green, stay out of

Colour preservation

- Use only products with low alcohol content.
- Wait at least a day before washing hair after colouring.
- Don't wash hair more often than is absolutely necessary.
- Avoid dry heat, chlorine, and direct sun exposure.
- Use a UV protection conditioner or spray.
- Don't perm and colour your hair on the same day.
- After shampooing, use a colour-enhancing conditioner created for your hair's hue.

chlorinated pools. Chlorine can react with the chemicals used to process hair, which can cause the colour to turn. It damages the structure of the hair and strips away natural oils. Wear a bathing cap and rinse your hair immediately after swimming. Clarifying formulas can also help correct a greenish hue. Use cool or lukewarm water when rinsing out your conditioner to help lock in colour and seal it in.

Blonde ambitions

You don't have to go lighter – the length and cut of your hair are what's really important – but virtually any woman who wants to try life as a blonde can. Even women with dark eyes, olive skin and dark brown hair can make the transition. If you're tempted to go golden, there has never been a better time.

The only way to lighten hair is bleaching. When you bleach your hair, hydrogen peroxide removes the natural pigment from the cortex first. Bleaching is permanent and roots will need to be touched up every 4–6 weeks. The next step is to add a rinse for a warm (reddish), cool (ashy) or neutral hue. Flat or one-dimensional blondes like platinum require more maintenance. Highlights and lowlights may be a better option. Highlights should complement your natural colour. Be wary of over highlighting that can leave your complexion looking drab and faded.

The sun naturally lightens the front of your hair, so don't add too many highlights to the back of your head to keep it looking natural. Lightening hair can also create a thicker appearance by matching the hair more closely to the scalp.

shades of grey

Perhaps the most dramatic age-related change that every woman eventually experiences is greying hair. Most women start to see grey from their early 30s to middle 40s.

For the most part, going grey is genetically determined – you may notice a change in colour around the same age as your mother. As you age, everything gets lighter as pigment fades, including your hair, which turns grey due to a lack of melanin pigment through decreased melanocyte function. This is irreversible. Blondes, redheads and light brunettes usually go grey, whereas those with darker brown and black hair are more likely to turn white.

Grey hair can take on a yellowish tinge from the effects of sun, wind and pollution. Colour-enhancing shampoos and conditioners can help cut brassy tints. Brightening shampoos prevent discolouration and add shine. Extra conditioning is needed for grey or white hair, which tends to be more coarse and dry. As the cortex goes, hair gets more wiry, dry and brittle, which can make it harder to manage. Use deep conditioners, leave-in lotions and silicone-based anti-frizz gels for taming. Shine products add lustre to greys, which can look dull and flat.

Nothing ages a woman faster than grey hair. Your choices are to keep the grey, cover it or let it gradually come in without taking over. To cover grey, hair can be dyed back to its original colour or slightly lighter. For partial coverage, semi-permanent colours can add a touch of silvery or slate tones. Permanent dyes conceal more grey. Lowlights can emphasize silver and grey by darkening selected strands of hair.

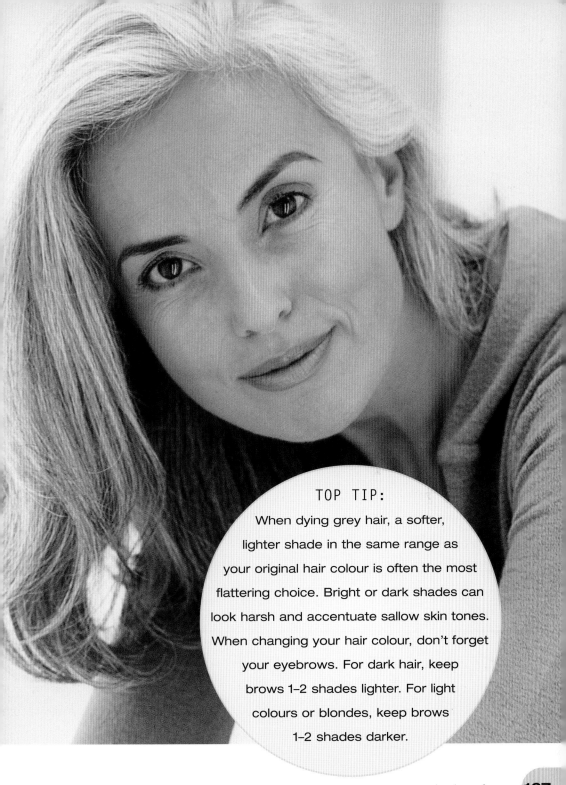

TOP TIP:

When dying grey hair, a softer, lighter shade in the same range as your original hair colour is often the most flattering choice. Bright or dark shades can look harsh and accentuate sallow skin tones. When changing your hair colour, don't forget your eyebrows. For dark hair, keep brows 1–2 shades lighter. For light colours or blondes, keep brows 1–2 shades darker.

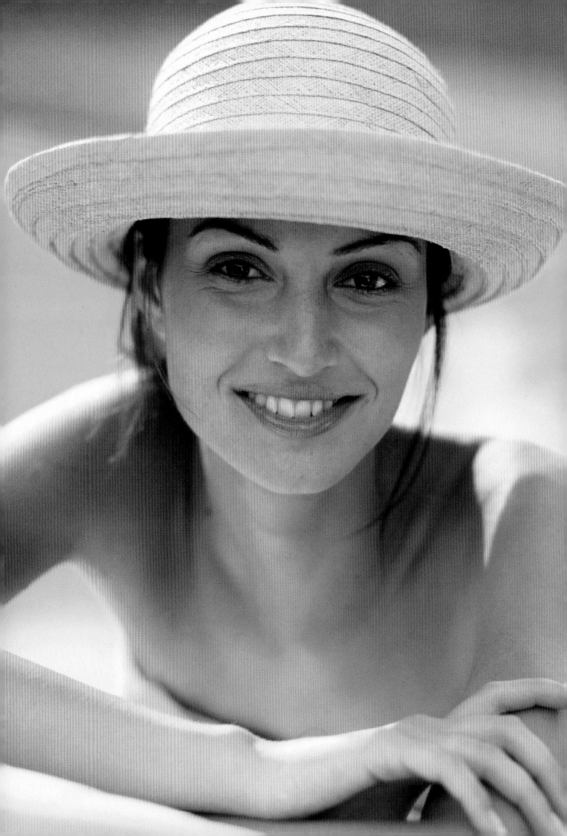

LOSING IT
LOSING IT

Being follically challenged is no laughing matter. Hair loss is a natural part of the ageing process, along with sagging necks, stained teeth, and wrinkles. Hair loss is often dismissed as another casualty on the road to getting older. While it can be the bane of your existence, thinning hair doesn't have to be the end of the world.

If you think you might be seeing a few extra hairs wedged between your bristles lately, you're not alone. Many women think thinning hair is a man's problem, but hair loss is more common in women than you think. For every 5 men with hereditary hair loss, there are 3 women experiencing the same condition. It can begin as early as your 20s and by the age of 35, almost 40 per cent of women demonstrate some of the signs. By the age of 50, half of all women experience some degree of hair thinning.

Women often miss the early signs, thinking that their hair is simply becoming finer. Putting off seeking medical attention to find out why your hair is thinning can make the difference between effective treatment and having to live with it. Although there are far more medical treatments available for men on the market, hair transplants can work wonders for women to fill out areas around the hair line and crown.

ages and stages

The life of the hair is similar to the life of the skin. In your 20s you love your hair, then somewhere in your fourth decade, your first grey hair arrives. At first there are only a few and they are easy to pluck out, but with each passing decade, the number of grey hairs increases.

20s Hair grows fastest from the age of 16–24 • Strands turn darker • Oil glands work overtime

30s First stray grey hairs appear • Hair starts to get finer • Hair needs extra protection from damage

40s Grey hairs are coming in fast and furious • There are now too many grey strays to pluck • Due to a reduction in oestrogen levels, hair thins and becomes drier and duller

50s The menopause and loss of oestrogen contribute to further hair loss • Your long hair days are over • Hormone fluctuations can make you lose hair from the top of your head and grow it on your face

60s Your hair has turned from grey to white • The oil glands have slowed down, making hair drier • Your hair continues to thin out

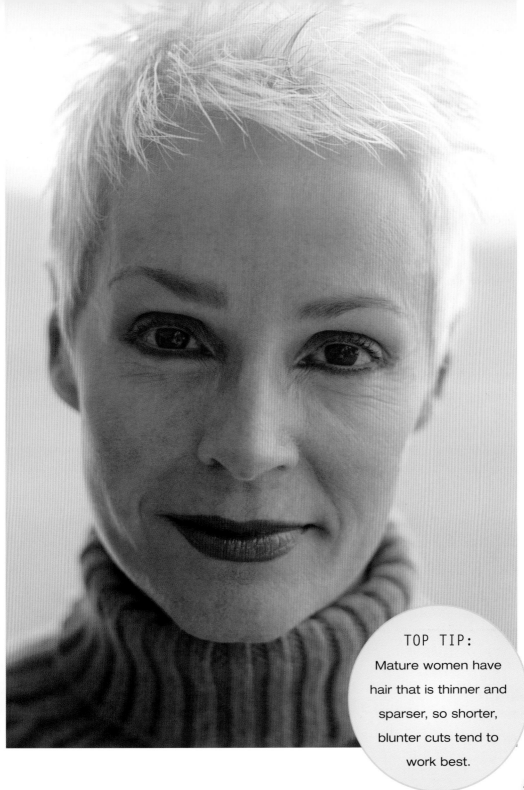

TOP TIP:
Mature women have hair that is thinner and sparser, so shorter, blunter cuts tend to work best.

thinning out of control

Hair is alive; it grows, it rests, it breaks, it dies and unfortunately it falls out. It sometimes grows back the same, less, or not at all.

The best way to keep it from falling out prematurely is to thicken what you've got from the inside out and to maintain its strength and condition. Finding hairs in your sink could just be your hair going through the usual process. If you are not on your way to balding, your hair will grow back just as strong. If you are, however, your hair will grow back finer and will not grow as long as it used to before falling out again. If the cause is largely genetic, topical medications may be a good place to start.

If you are suffering from excessive hair loss, before setting off on a search for wigs or hair transplants, your first step should be a consultation with a dermatologist to determine the cause. It is best to begin treatment in the early stages, when you first begin to display signs of hair loss. As with any medical condition, hair loss responds better to treatment if caught early.

Rooting out the cause is key

Female hair loss can be difficult to diagnose, as different conditions have a similar appearance. Causes range from genetics, hormonal flux, poor circulation, stress, rapid weight loss, and certain medications. The doctor will take a detailed medical history and

TOP TIP:
Female pattern hair loss can begin in the late teens to 20s, and can progress if left untreated.

possibly perform diagnostic tests to determine the cause of your hair loss. There are some health conditions that can go undetected, which contribute to hair loss. For example, an underactive or overactive thyroid gland and iron deficiency can cause shedding. Hair loss could be the first sign of a medical problem, so don't ignore it.

Diagnostic tests

Thyroid function tests: Checking the thyroid-stimulating hormone to rule out thyroid abnormalities.

Blood tests: Studies to measure blood lipids, complete blood count (CBC).

Hormone levels: DHEAS, testosterone, androstenedione, prolactin, follicular stimulating hormone, leutinizing hormone, to identify hormonal conditions.

Iron deficiencies: Serum iron, serum ferritin, total iron binding capacity (TIBC), to rule out anaemia.

Venereal Disease Research Laboratory Test (VDRL): A test to rule out syphilis, a disease that can cause patchy hair loss.

After carefully examining the scalp and hair, further tests may be needed as a screening mechanism to determine general health, as well as specific abnormalities that may contribute to hair thinning. Once the underlying cause is identified – if one can be pinpointed – it should be treated. For example, if you have a thyroid condition, thyroid-replacement hormones may be prescribed. Women with heavy menstrual periods can develop an iron deficiency due to blood loss. If you have low serum iron, iron pills may be recommended.

getting the shaft

getting the shaft

There can be many reasons why your hair may be falling out; genetics, stress, diet, hormones and chemicals. Some of these may be entirely out of your control.

The most common cause of thinning is heredity. Hair loss can be passed down from either your mother's or your father's side of the family. The more bald people there are in your family, the greater your chances of losing your hair. Contrary to common belief, it does not skip a generation. The propensity is passed down from any and all of your relatives. About half the people who have one balding parent of either sex will inherit the dominant gene for baldness.

FOLLICLE FACT:
Balding is predominant among Caucasians and more common in those with fine hair.

Hormonal flux

Periods of hormonal change are a common cause of female hair loss. Women can lose hair after pregnancy, following discontinuation of birth control pills or during the menopause. The changes that occur during pregnancy usually slow down the shedding process, which is why some women's hair becomes nice and thick. But within a few months of childbirth, the hair that did not get shed during pregnancy seems to fall out all at once. Hair loss may not show up for 3 months after hormonal flux and it may take another 3 months for the normal growth pattern to resume.

Diet details

By their very nature, crash diets can cause temporary hair loss by putting stress on your system. Protein or iron deficiencies may affect your hair count. Many over-the-counter diet supplements contain high doses of vitamin A, which may worsen thinning. Rapid or sudden weight loss can also contribute.

Tress stress

Surgery, severe illness and emotional stress can have a negative impact on your hair. The body can simply shut down the production of hair during periods of stress, and devotes its energies towards repairing vital body structures. There may be a 3 month delay between the onset of stress and the first signs of hair loss. There may be another 3 month delay before the return of noticeable hair regrowth. Although they will not cause balding on their own, physical and emotional stress can adversely affect the quality and strength of the hair. Stress does not cause permanent hair loss.

One of the most common complaints women have after a facelift or forehead (brow) lift is hair thinning, specifically along the sides of the head. The cause is often the tension the stitches or staples place on the hair follicles. Modified facelifts are designed to avoid making any incisions in the hairline for this reason. Post surgery hair loss is usually a temporary condition and regrowth occurs within the first 3–4 months. If you are already experiencing thinning hair and are contemplating a lift, talk to your surgeon to determine your risk level. Some cosmetic surgeons may recommend using a course of Minoxidil (see page 182) before and after surgery as a precaution. Use it twice daily for a period of 4 months for best results.

girl stuff

The most common type of hair loss in women is androgenetic alopecia, also known as female pattern baldness. This involves thinning of the hair over the top and sides of the head.

Women lose their hair differently to men: it's usually less severe and most commonly seen after the menopause, although it can begin as early as puberty. Unlike men, who tend to lose hair in a concentrated area, women are prone to overall thinning, which starts at the top, gradually spreads and the scalp may become visible. Women can also have male pattern baldness – a receding hairline and bald spot at the crown. Androgenetic alopecia can lead to a progressive miniaturisation of hair follicles and shortening of the hair growth cycle. The active growth phase becomes shorter and the hair follicles smaller, so the follicles produce finer hairs. Eventually there is no growth at all.

Alopecia areata is the second most common form of hair loss, although mostly temporary. Follicles stop producing hair abruptly. At its mildest, small patches appear where less than 50 per cent of scalp hair is lost; the most severe form involves more than half of all scalp hair. Alopecia totalis is the complete loss of scalp hair and alopecia universalis involves the total loss of all body hair. Other types of temporary hair loss include anagen effluvium, mainly due to internally administered medications, such as chemotherapy agents, and telogen effluvium, when more than the usual number of follicles enter the resting stage.

BEAUTY BYTE:
To learn about hair loss in women, log on to www.womenshairinstitute.com.

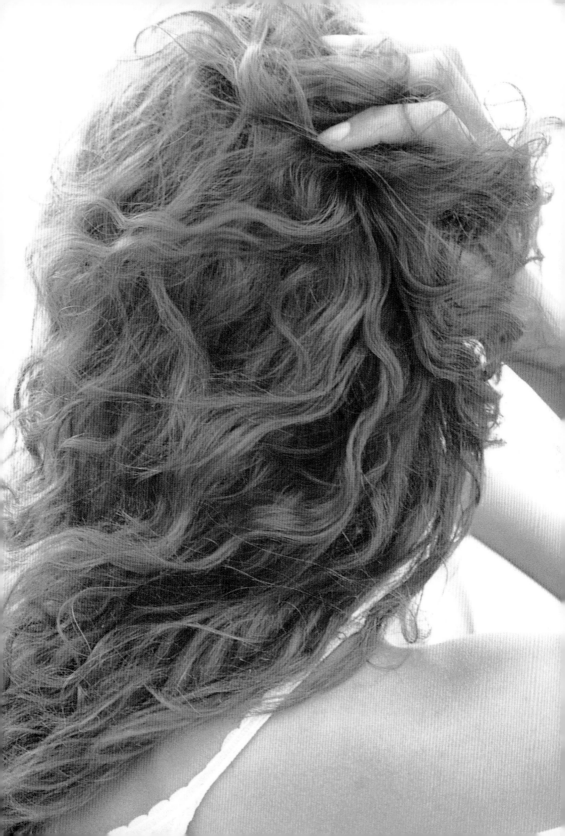

fuzz busters

Getting rid of unsightly hair on your underarms, bikini line, legs and arms can be a religious experience. DIY methods are an alternative to expensive salon or clinic therapies.

The rate of hair growth can change with age and varies from person to person. Body and facial hair is always growing, just as the hair on your head grows. Women's facial hair typically grows to a maximum of 3mm. Leg and body hair can grow longer, up to about 13mm. Women's leg hair primarily grows in one direction: down. Women's underarm hair grows in all directions. Women's underarm hair grows about twice as fast as leg hair.

Shaving is the most popular way to remove hair, and the cheapest and quickest. Regrowth shows up with a blunt, rather than a tapered end, so it can feel coarser. Most women have to shave every day to stay smooth. Waxing is the longest-lasting temporary hair removal technique available. When wax is warm, it enters the follicle, allowing the hair to be pulled out from the root. Hair grows back in 3–6 weeks. Waxing makes your hair grow back lighter over time. A transparent wax lets you see the hairs that have been covered and determine the direction of their growth. Hair must be at least 4mm before waxing.

Depilatory creams work by penetrating the hair shaft, dissolving If you seek more permanent hair reduction, the best choices are electrolysis, lasers and light sources. For long-term hair removal, the follicle has to be obliterated along with its root. Electrolysis destroys the root through the use of a thin metal probe that is slid into a follicle, through which electricity is delivered which causes localised damage.

'Permanent' is often an illusion, but staying hair free for up to 2 years with lasers is possible. Light energy converts to heat as it passes through the skin and is absorbed by the melanin in the follicle. When the temperature reaches a high enough level in a hair follicle during its active phase, the targeted hair structures are destroyed which inhibits re-growth. On sensitive areas like underarms and bikini zone you may feel a sharp stinging. The more potent the laser, the more it hurts, but the more hairs zapped in one go. A cooling gel is a must.

There are many systems on the market, and all of them work to some degree. Among the most popular technologies are the Diode laser and Intense Pulsed Light devices (IPLs). IPLs use a broad spectrum of light to treat a variety of hair and skin colours and hair depths. Most systems target pigment, so dark hairs on light skin is the best combination. Light hair on light skin doesn't work as well. Possible side effects include scarring, burns, redness and swelling, and darker skin types are more at risk. Thousands of hairs can be zapped in a single treatment session which works well for large areas like the back, arms and legs. Long-lasting laser hair removal typically requires multiple treatments, which can be costly. Regrowth between treatments comes in thinner and finer.

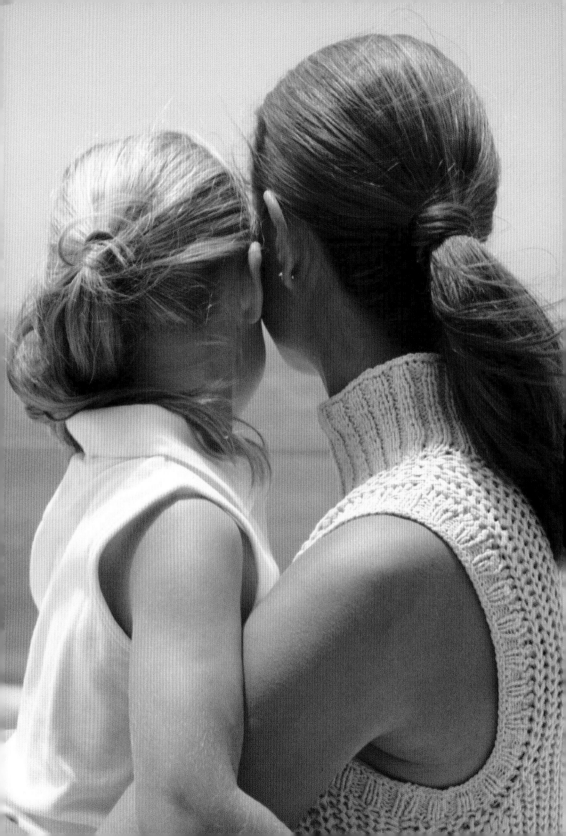

RESTORING IT

RESTORING IT

Having a hair transplant may never occur to many women, since it is usually thought of as something reserved for men. Gone are the days when transplants made a scalp look like a field of newly planted corn. Large grafting procedures that gave transplants their plug-like appearance are a thing of the past. The new methods allow for more hairs in each graft, to be placed between existing hairs, promoting greater hair density.

Mini- and micrografts, along with mega-sessions and Follicular Unit Hair Transplants (FUHT) gained acceptance in the 1990s and remain popular due to their natural appearance. Today transplants can correct and enhance your natural hairline and be virtually undetectable.

The future of hair transplanting may lie in using a flexible robotic arm, which has two video cameras mounted on to it to take a three-dimensional image of your head. The arm is anchored to a table and can be programmed to extract the follicular units and dramatically speed up what is now a very tedious process.

For women not too keen to go under the knife, glamourous hair extensions can instantly create fullness and length that would take years to grow on your own. These methods are high maintenance and pricey, but results can be Hollywood hair.

great pretenders

great pretenders

If you don't have the patience to wait for your hair to grow or if your hair, when long, looks stringy rather than luscious, consider hair extensions.

Extensions come in all sizes, textures and colours. Lasting for weeks, the swatch of hair – either synthetic or human (costly, but worth it) – can be stitched, braided, glued or woven into your hair. As extensions are not part of your natural hairline, you need to take a few extra steps. First, cleanse your scalp thoroughly and shampoo gently. Use a soft bristle brush and start from the bottom, gently working your way up to avoid pulling out your extensions. Sleep with your hair tied up and never go to bed with it wet. For braided extensions, run your fingers through the braids to prevent tangles; do not spray braids with conditioners or any silicone-based products, as they will slip. If you want to colour, curl or set extensions, go to a salon or you might risk damaging your scalp and hair. Most extensions last about 3 months when they fall out. For a temporary effect, use DIY clip-on hair extensions; attach them close to the scalp so your hair hides them.

If your hair is thinning to the point that emergency measures are needed, a hairpiece can give you a good match to your own colour. Women with thinning hair often choose partial hair additions. Hair weaving and other attachments can place prolonged tension that can cause permanent hair loss at the anchor site. Newer models are designed to minimise the potential for damage. For the most natural look, extensions should match your own hair in colour and texture and be no more than twice the length of your hair.

archery

Choosing the right brow shape is akin to choosing the right spectacles – they frame your face. Brows with an unnatural shape fight with the rest of your features.

You may need several good shapings to whip brows back into shape and in harmony with your face. Great brows are as close as you can get to an eyelift without the stitches. At their worst, they can really detract from your looks.

- If your brows have been over-tweezered, grow them out.

- The brow's incline should always be longer than the decline and its inner edge should line up with the inside edge of the nostril.

- The peak of the arch and the outer end of the brow should sit along an imaginary line drawn from the tip of the nose through the pupil to the peak of the arch, and through the eye's outer corner to the end of the brow.

- Avoid plucking too much from the inner brow.

- Your inner brow should be no thinner than the radius of your iris, to keep the brow from looking too surprised.

- Never fill in brows with too dark a colour, even for very dark or black brows. Use fine strokes to lightly fill in skimpy spots.

- Thick brows may be overpowering and make eyes look smaller.

- No face is perfectly symmetrical; it is common to have one brow slightly higher or lower or a different shape from the other.

hair growth stimulators

Minoxidil is the only FDA-approved drug to treat female hair loss. Most other prescription medication is used only for men.

Minoxidil

Topical Minoxidil, marketed under the brand name Regaine, is currently the only medication approved by the US FDA for female-pattern hair loss. Minoxidil is often more effective for women than men. This anti-balding drug is a topical ointment applied directly to the scalp twice daily. It increases blood flow to the scalp, which has been associated with increased hair growth. More potent formulas can be obtained through a doctor but it can cause irritation and itchiness in higher doses. The downside is that it has to be used continually to maintain hair growth, and takes about 4 months to see results. If you stop, the normal hair loss process will start again and you will lose your newly regrown hair in 3–4 months. Regaine is not a cure for baldness but it can slow down the hair loss process and help you retain the hair you have. If you get regrowth, it's an added bonus, but there is no guarantee. Some doctors will combine progesterone with Minoxidil to boost its effects.

The best hope for women short of transplant surgery lies in the area of hormone treatments. Oestrogens compete with androgens for control over the body. Hair loss may be helped by raising the ratio of female to male hormones. Some doctors prescribe topical and oral oestrogen for hair thinning, especially in post-menopausal women.

Anti-androgens

Spironolactone is a drug known as an androgen blocker. An increased amount of androgens or an increased sensitivity of androgen receptors play a major role in hairloss in both men and women. Spironolactone blocks androgen receptors that decrease the amount of hormone activity in women. It takes 3-6 months to see results. Other anti-androgens that are used for hairloss include cyproterone acetate. These drugs are also used to treat acne, overactive oil glands and hirsutism (excessive hair growth). Studies have shown that palmetto may act in a similar way, but it has yet to be proven as a treatment for hair loss.

Finasteride and Dutasteride

Finasteride (Propecia) is a tablet taken once daily that has been shown to help preserve exisiting hair in men. This pill blocks the conversion of testosterone into a hormone called dihydrotestosterone (DHT), which converts normal hair follicles to non-hair follicles causing hairloss. Dustasteride is a newer medication that works in a similar way. These drugs are not generally recommended for women of childbearing age.

Hope in a soap

There are a number of shampoos, conditioners and serums that promote a variety of theories on preventing hair loss. Some systems contain deep-cleansing agents that open up clogged follicles, allowing these tiny sacs to sprout new hair shafts. These products may be effective as scalp conditioners and make hair appear healthier, but they do little, if anything, to reverse hair loss.

hair restorers

hair restorers

What you see in the mirror over a period of time is the best sign of early thinning. You may notice areas of hair that no longer need cutting or where the hairs are shorter and finer.

Trichologists administer non-medical treatments for scalp and hair problems. The term simply means 'hair specialist' and carries no specific training or licencing. Typically, a qualified trichologist will have completed an educational programme that covers the anatomy and physiology of the skin and hair. During an initial consultation the trichologist will analyse both hair and scalp under a microscope to determine the problem and best way to treat it.

Dermatologists are trained in the knowledge and treatment of hair loss, but not all dermatologists specialise in medical or surgical treatments. There is a wide range in the quality of hair replacement surgery, which can run from really obvious to virtually undetectable. Through the use of variable-sized grafts and improved instrumentation, experienced hair restoration surgeons can create a natural hair appearance by lowering a receding hairline and filling in thinning areas at the temples and crown with precision. Find out about a surgeon's qualifications. Typically, hair restoration surgery is performed by dermatologists and plastic surgeons, although general surgeons often perform these procedures. Make sure your surgeon has extensive experience and training and does a lot of hair restoration procedures on a consistent, ongoing basis. Practice makes perfect.

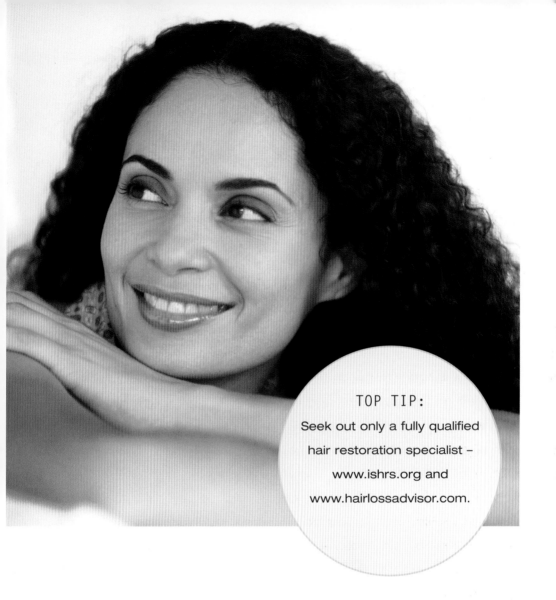

TOP TIP:

Seek out only a fully qualified

hair restoration specialist –

www.ishrs.org and

www.hairlossadvisor.com.

Caveat emptor: Before you sign on the dotted line, be wary of hair restoration clinics that ask you to pay in advance for extensive programs without any written guarantee of results. Expect to pay a consultation fee, and if treatment is recommended, ask to pay at the time of the treatment. Clinics will sometimes offer a free consultation to induce you to come in.

hair lines

Although there is an abundance of so-called remedies for baldness in a bottle, the only way to restore your hairline is to get help from a hair restoration specialist.

Hair transplantation, formerly one of the most tedious and labour-intensive cosmetic surgery procedures, is now a simple day surgery done under local anaesthetic. The best method depends on the extent and pattern of hair loss. Often a combination of techniques will be needed. The ideal candidate for hair transplants is a woman who has either female-pattern or male-pattern baldness and enough hair on the back of the head to redistribute to where it is thinning. Female pattern baldness is progressive; the results you get today may not stay that way, so your surgeon has to plan your hairline and the density of transplanted hair for the long term.

Women are considered more challenging to treat for hair loss than men. As in most things, our expectations are higher. In a man, if he sees he has a little more on top and maybe looks a few years younger, he's usually satisfied. Women want thick, glossy hair all the time. Hair transplants can actually be simpler for women because they're able to hide them better. Because women's hair is generally longer, it's harder to see the incision. When new hair begins to grow, the effect on a woman's scalp is more subtle. People may notice that your hair looks better but they won't be quite sure why. Something else to be aware of is that transplanting hairs next to existing hairs can bring on traumatic shock, which causes existing hairs to shed. This can lead you to actually look worse after a procedure than before. The shock loss is usually temporary, but since the existing hairs may also be damaged by pattern loss, it is possible they won't grow back. If the transplant is done carefully, so as not to disturb the existing hairs, it won't induce shock loss.

Hair transplants are like plant cuttings. The technique moves your own hair follicles from the back or side of the head and transplants them to the thinning or balding areas, where they will regrow naturally. Done well, it can look very natural. After all, it's your own naturally growing hair. Small donor strips of hair-bearing scalp are removed from the back and sides of the head, which is an area of the densest hair for even the baldest heads. The area that grafts are taken from is called the 'donor site'. The beauty of the methods used today is that only ONE fine white scar in the back of the scalp is necessary. The surgeon can keep using the same hidden scar over and over for any transplant procedures that may be needed in the future. The strips of scalp are divided into grafts for placement in the balding areas. The hair-bearing grafts are carefully inserted into small holes or slits that are made in the balding scalp. The grafts can also be inserted between existing hairs to increase the density and thicken the area.

Strategic planning and precise placement of grafts is essential to give the illusion of more hair.

REALITY CHECK:
Approximately one-third of women with thinning hair are candidates for hair transplants.

mini- & micrografts

Mini- and micrografts are the most commonly performed hair procedures for women, and remain the treatment of choice.

The characteristics of your hair and scalp – colour, texture, skin-to-scalp contrast, hair density, degree of curl, estimated future hair loss and amount of donor hair – determine whether you are a good candidate for a graft. Over the last decade, the basic size of hair grafts has become smaller and finer. Micrografts as small as single hairs are commonly placed behind the hairline to provide a gradually increasing density. They are ideal to fill in the hairline region, a common problem area for women. Most surgeons use a combination of variable-sized grafts for the most natural-looking results.

Micrograft: 1–2 hairs into needle holes.

Small slit grafts: 3–4 hairs into a slit recipient site.

Large slit grafts: 5–7 hairs into a slit recipient site.

Small minigraft: 3–4 hairs into a small recipient site.

Large minigraft: 5–8 hairs into a small round recipient site.

It is now possible to move about 400–500 skin grafts of 2–4 hairs each from the back of the head to the front and top in one session. Initially the donor hair falls out within a few weeks, but regrows 3 months later. Within 4–6 months, you see a huge difference, and it continues to grow for as long as the hair would have done

BEAUTY BYTES:

For more information, log on to www.ahlc.org, www.hairlossdirect.com

had it been left in the site from which it was removed. Transplants are labour intensive and require the skill of a surgeon along with a team of 3–5 assistants. Mega-sessions can deliver 3,000–4,000 grafts, taking 10–12 hours and involving several technicians. The amount of density that you can achieve depends on the number of grafts placed per session. Most women only require 1 or 2 treatment sessions for a good correction. In some cases the holes or slits needed to reposition hair follicles can be made with the aid of laser technology. The laser creates very small punctures of a consistent depth and width, which in some cases can speed up the length of time the procedure takes. It causes less bleeding and incurs a shorter healing time.

Gene therapy

Recombinant DNA gene therapy is the most likely prospect as a cure for baldness. Researchers have pinpointed the first human gene linked to baldness, which may provide key information on how hair grows. It may eventually be possible to give you back the gene that codes you for a particular deficiency. Creams that contain the gene may be developed so it can be transferred via the body into the bloodstream. Topical creams could also be applied directly to the hair follicle. Cloning scientists are currently working on hair cloning – a tissue-engineering technique that uses a single hair follicle to create thousands more, which can then be inserted into a bald area of the scalp. Growing new hair follicles from existing ones could actually increase the number of hairs on your head, instead of just repositioning them as hair replacements do.

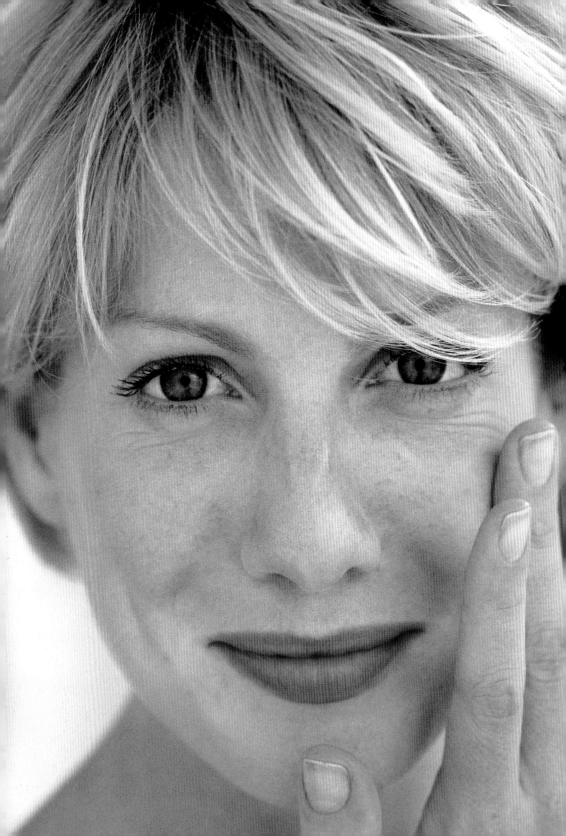

WRINKLE RESCUE

WRINKLE RESCUE

We all age, but looking older is a matter of choice. Wrinkles form largely because levels of collagen — a component of the connective tissue in the skin that creates flexibility — decrease over time. The two major ways skin ages are: intrinsic ageing, which is genetically programmed and affects the skin all over your body; and photoageing, resulting from the long-term effects of sun, smoking and pollution. The degree to which skin ages is also determined genetically to some extent. Fair-skinned people tend to age more and earlier than those with darker skin types that are pigment protected.

The earlier you start caring for your complexion, the better it will serve you long term. Anti-wrinkle treatments can undo damage, but prevention is best. 80 per cent of the lines you see in the mirror were caused by the sun. The other 20 per cent result from smiling, pouting, chatting and frowning — any facial movements. It is never too late to start preventing new wrinkles, or to soften the ones you have.

There is a virtual smorgasbord of topical wrinkle remedies and non-surgical treatments available for the scalpel shy to choose from. Nothing yet can replace a facelift or eye lift, but you can stay looking younger for longer without surgery. Once your neck and jowls are your biggest concern, it's time to think about a facelift.

face facts

The skin that gets exposed to those nasty UV rays the most – your face, neck and hands – will age fastest.

Skin that is the thinnest on the body, like the delicate eyelid area, is most susceptible to damage, lines, and ageing. Thinning skin is a result of a breakdown of collagen fibres. Skin loses elasticity, especially if it has been exposed to sunlight and becomes fragile. Skin dries out because the structure weakens and it doesn't retain moisture as well as younger skin. With menopause comes declining oestrogen levels. Skin usually gets drier. However some women become oilier even if they never had oily skin as a teenager.

Most wrinkle creams are oil-based and work by blocking the release of water from the skin. As it ages, skin loses the ability to attract moisture and fundamentally becomes dehydrated. The amount of natural lubrication or sebum produced declines so it needs to be replenished in order to attract and retain water. The drier your skin is, the heavier the moisturiser you need. However, not every complexion needs a daily application of moisturiser. If your skin is oily, you need less. Moisturising is like a savings plan with the benefits only showing after time.

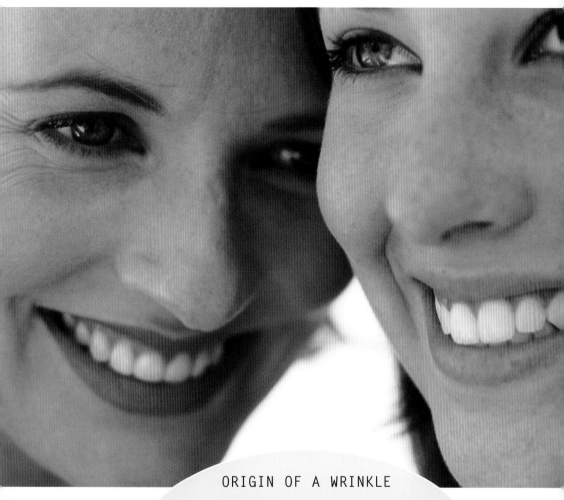

ORIGIN OF A WRINKLE

Fine wrinkles: Caused by the breakdown of collagen and elastin fibres over time.

Deep wrinkles: Caused by the building up of muscle in the deep layers below the surface of the skin.

Dynamic wrinkles: Only visible when muscles are engaged, as in smiling or frowning.

Static wrinkles: Seen all the time, when the face is at rest or moving.

skin ageing

So you think your skin is going to look young forever. Guess again! At 30, it takes on a life of its own. Your mission is to outsmart your skin cells before they get the better of you.

20s **Skin heaven:** Your skin is clear of spots, your pores are invisible and your complexion is even and taut. Save your skin by using an SPF 15 every day and getting your tan out of a bottle, tube or spray. Start your preventive anti-ageing regime with a good eye cream to hold off crow's-feet. Cleanse well, remove all traces of dirt and make-up before going to bed and keep oil plugs at bay with good exfoliation.

30s **Party's over:** Expect to see visible changes in your skin's texture. This can be a real eye opener. Cell turnover gently slows down, so adding exfoliants to speed it up is key. It's the perfect time to start more intense anti-ageing skin care. Collagen and elastin fibres begin to break down, so keep them firm by integrating nutrients into your programme like Vitamin C, AHAs, antioxidants, and plant enzymes. Smokers will start to see fine lines around the mouth and squinters will spy their first crow's-feet. It's the perfect time to start non-invasive anti-wrinkle treatments like Botox, peels and lasers for thread veins.

40s   **They're here:** Your wrinkles are in full force, so it's time to bring out the heavy artillery. Everything becomes lazy: Skin gets drier, and sagging and wrinkles give way to folds, furrows, and creases. Your brow droops and the corners of your mouth turn down as jowls creep up. The best plan is to fight back with medically advanced skin-care formulas which are worth spending money on. Look for high-tech ingredients like antioxidants and enzymes, which should keep your face and neck supple. Wage war on brown spots with lightening agents. Continue a regime of peels, Botox, and wrinkle fillers to combat creases. This is the ideal time to start considering surgical options (eye, face and brow lifts) to plan your beauty future.

50s   **Desperate measures:** It's a big number, but don't let it get you down. Turn back the clock with rejuvenating treatments, firming masks and moisturising serums. Your hormones are wreaking havoc, accounting for enlarged pores and increased oil activity. At this stage, you will get limited results from para-surgical treatments. Once your jawline starts to soften and the nasal labial folds require lots of filling, the time has come to nip or tuck. Face and neck lift techniques have come a long way. With shorter scars and faster healing, they are the mainstay in a woman's arsenal against ageing. By having your first lift before you turn 50, you may never have to go public. It won't make you look 25 again, but it can keep your big birthday a secret for longer.

skin care jungle

Examine your face and let that be your guide. Your skin looks different every day, so adjust your skin care accordingly. Delete or substitute products and treatments as needed.

The factors that determine how long your skin will stay glowing include genetics, diet and nutrition, sun exposure, smoking and drinking, and stress levels. The best defense is to protect your skin from free-radicals and use therapies that go on a search-and-destroy mission to neutralise them. Repairing skin with visible signs of ageing will not happen overnight. It is like beginning an exercise programme – start slow, gradually increasing your tolerance in stages. If you stop, the problem comes back again. Every woman is constantly looking for the perfect skin care regime; a cleanser that removes make-up and leaves skin feeling comfortable, a toner that refreshes without drying and a moisturiser that hydrates without clogging pores. A great skin care regime involves more than one miracle product and varies from one face to another.

Hot water and soap dissolve the skin's natural moisture, so keep your daily shower short and water temperature moderate. While bathing, rub your body with a washcloth to exfoliate. Gently pat yourself dry. While the skin is still damp, apply a moisturiser. In general, the heavier the moisturiser, the better it works on dry skin. When the skin becomes dry, it needs water to help rejuvenate it, and moisturisers trap water in the skin. Relief for dry skin typically comes in these forms: ointments, creams, oils, and lotions.

Ointments are thick, greasy and best at preventing moisture escaping from the skin. Ointments are best for areas that take a lot of abuse, such as hands, elbows, and feet. Creams are heavier than lotions and more effective at trapping moisture in normal to dry skin. Oils are easily absorbed when applied to slightly damp skin after you pat dry, but often less moisturising than ointments, creams, or lotions. Lotions are thinner and lighter so are least effective at replacing lost moisture in very dry skin, but can be applied and absorbed easily. They are good for normal, oily, and young skin that doesn't need much hydration. Lotions are also good for the body, but are less effective at sealing moisture in than ointments or creams. Some face and neck formulas will be too heavy around the eyes. If your eyes are puffy, use a lighter formula. Thick creams may trap too much moisture in the skin and cause swelling.

Cleanse (and tone): Use a gentle, non-detergent cleanser and make sure to rinse off all residue. You only need a toner if your skin doesn't feel clean without it, you are in a humid climate or have oily or acne-prone skin.

Exfoliate: All skins need some form of exfoliation, but the degree will differ.

Treat: This phase encompasses everything from treating acne and eczema and bleaching dark spots to oil control and anti-ageing.

Moisturise: Skin needs hydration, but not all skin needs the same amount. Oily skin needs less or none in particularly pimple-prone areas. The eyelid area needs more because it has the fewest oil glands.

Protect: Every skin needs UVA/UVB protection daily with a minimum SPF 15, all year long.

TOP TIP:
A haphazard approach to skin care is destined to fail. Take the time to get educated and don't be afraid to get help from a professional.

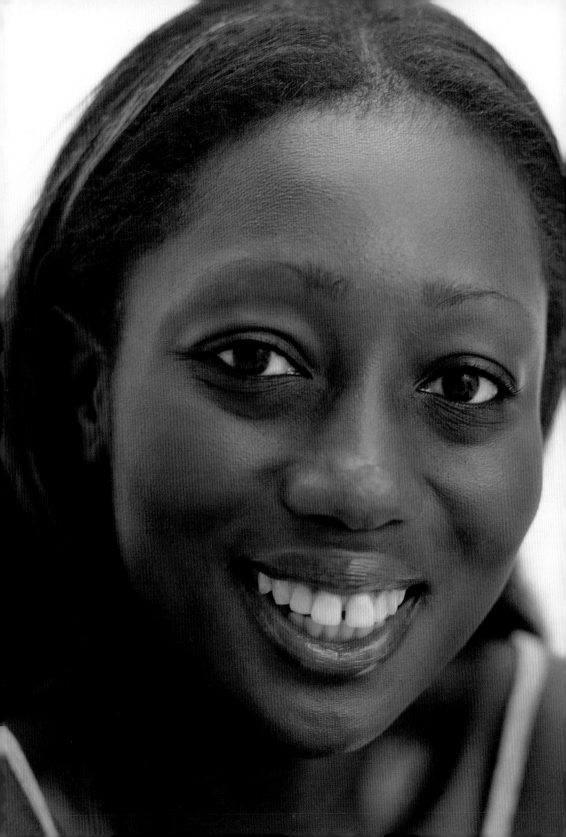

PREVENTING THEM

PREVENTING THEM

An ounce of prevention is worth a pound of cure in future wrinkle remedies. The best way to deal with wrinkles is not to get them in the first place. Protecting the skin from the sun is the single most important part of caring for it. Continuous sun exposure wrinkles and dries out the skin, leaving it coarse and thick. Uneven pigmentation, freckles, and dark patches are also side effects. The earliest warning sign of severe damage is the development of 'actinic keratoses'. These pre-cancerous lesions are most common in people with fair skin and light hair, but can affect any skin type. If left untreated, AK's can turn into deadly forms of skin cancer.

As you age cumulative sun damage will start to crop up when you least suspect it. The sun's rays are very unforgiving, and the damage they do to the skin is inescapable. Products used for prevention don't necessarily produce visible results. For example, your sunscreen won't reduce wrinkles, but consistent use will keep them from forming as quickly and as deeply.

The first step in a programme to revise the signs of ageing should be the introduction of the new generation of 'cosmeceuticals', which, by definition, are cosmetics that exert a pharmacologic effect on the skin.

ray bans

Approximately 5 per cent of the UV radiation hitting the skin is reflected. The remaining 95 per cent passes into the tissue, gets scattered and then passes out again, or gets absorbed by molecules in the various layers of the epidermis and dermis.

How wrinkled your skin gets depends largely on how much sun you have been exposed to in your lifetime. People who spend a lot of time outside without adequate protection develop leathery skin earlier, which makes them look older than they are. To judge the effects of the sun on your skin, compare the appearance of your hands to that of any sun protected skin. Start protecting your skin early, preferably while your still in nappies. Up to 50 per cent of your total UV radiation exposure is acquired by the age of 18, and 75 per cent by the age of 30.

Light spectrum

The longer the wavelength, the greater the energy level and the more damage it can do.

UVA are longer wavelengths, mostly transmitted to the dermis where they cause damage in the deeper skin layers, and skin cancer.
UVB are shorter wavelengths, largely removed in the epidermis, particularly by DNA and melanin, and known to cause sunburn and skin cancer.

Free radicals make the difference between 'peaches 'n' cream' and 'wrinkled prune'. UV radiation has many effects on the skin as a result of its absorption by skin molecules, like DNA. After UV absorption, DNA undergoes chemical changes. If these alterations are not repaired, they can be disruptive to the way cells function. Even small amounts of sunlight on the skin can cause DNA damage throughout the entire thickness of the epidermis. Because UVB is largely absorbed high up before it reaches the dermis, most of the immediate damage is to the epidermis. Skin thickness increases with age, while skin elasticity decreases. The epidermis becomes more fragile. The melanocytes also stop functioning which causes brown spots, blotchiness or a sallow hue. These changes combine to make up visible skin ageing.

If your photoageing clock has been ticking for some time, minimise further changes by being careful from now on. Photoageing steadily develops even if you are simply taking a walk around the block or sitting at a street café. The skin doesn't need to turn red, pink, or burn for permanent damage to take place. Sunburn is a skin-repair process. Tanning is the release of UV-protective pigment following UV-induced DNA damage. Accumulated damage over many years produces deep wrinkles. Practising 'safe sun' and avoiding tanning beds are a MUST. The only safe tan is a fake tan. Tanning salons are Public Enemy #1 and a wrinkle's best friend.

REALITY CHECK:
Longer UVA and UVB wavelengths can pass through the atmosphere even on a cloudy day. They also penetrate car windows and sunglasses.

save your skin

save your skin

The incidence of skin cancer is growing at an alarming rate, making it the single most common form of cancer today. Sun exposure is universally cited as the primary cause of skin cancers because UV rays damage DNA cells.

Most cancerous lesions occur on body parts that are exposed to sunlight, like the face, neck, arms, legs and chest. Skin cancer is the uncontrollable growth of abnormal cells in a layer of the skin. It comes in many shapes, sizes and colours. The three major types have names that are all too familiar: Basal Cell Carcinoma, the most common form, usually looks like raised, translucent lumps or growths; Squamous Cell Carcinoma is characterised by crusty or scaly reddish patches, which can spread to other areas of the body; Malignant Melanoma is the least common but the most deadly form of skin cancer. It can look like a dark mole or blemish, ranges from brownish to black and can spread through the bloodstream and the lymphatic system. 'Actinic Keratoses' are dry, crusty, flaky, often brown or pink rough patches appearing on the face, hands, lips or elsewhere. These lesions signal that the sun has damaged the skin and are considered a precursor to skin cancer that one in six people will develop in their lifetime. Left untreated, they can develop into any form of skin cancer.

REALITY CHECK:
Any lesions bigger than 6mm should be checked by your doctor.

If detected and treated early, skin cancer has a cure rate of over 90 per cent. Without treatment, any skin cancer can cause serious damage and even death. When detected early, there are many effective treatment options. The biopsy is usually the first step. Cancerous growths can be surgically removed and excised, scraped away and treated with liquid nitrogen to freeze the tissue. Lasers can also be used to vaporise cancerous tissue in the layers of the skin and reduce pre-cancerous lesions like actinic keratoses. Topical agents are also used for very small basal cell carcinomas.

Never too early to start

Skin self-examinations should consist of regularly looking over your entire body, including your back, scalp, soles of feet, between your toes and the palms of your hands. To do a thorough examination, use a full-length mirror and a hand-held mirror so you can literally see behind you or ask your partner for assistance. Any changes in size, colour, shape or texture of an existing mole, the development of a new mole or any other unusual changes in the skin should be brought to the attention of your doctor. According to the British Association of Dermatologists, in at least 4 out of 5 cases, skin cancer is a preventable disease.

SIGNS OF PHOTOAGEING

- Dehydrated and thickened outer skin layers
- Flaking and rough skin
- Age spots and sunburn freckles
- Sallow complexion
- Enlarged pores clogged with sebum
- Broken, enlarged capillaries
- Milia or small white cysts

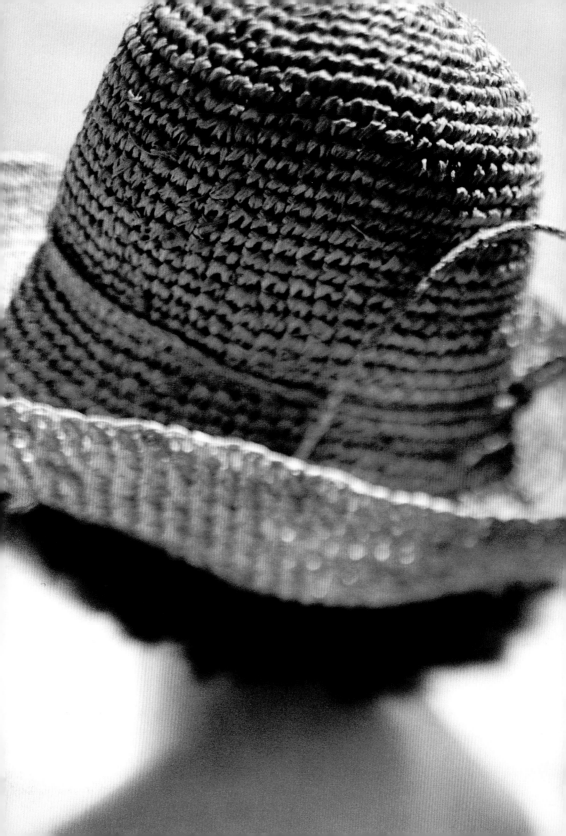

SPF savvy

Sunscreens temporarily absorb UV rays. The best formulas protect against both UVA – the culprit in wrinkle formation – and UVB, which causes tanning and burning.

The higher the Sun Protection Factor (SPF) rating, the stronger and longer its effects. The SPF index only addresses UVB rays. For protection against UVAs, look for broad spectrum products.

TOP TIP:
When it comes to sunscreen, rub it on, rub it in well, rub it all over and rub it on often.

The burning question is 'how much do I really need?' Sunblock should come in a six-pack, because most of us use far too little to be effective. Use sunscreen every day, all year round. Autumn and winter are no exception, no matter where you live or travel to. More sensitive skin types may tolerate physical blockers better. Sunscreens with a heavier coating provide a better physical barrier.

Screen versus block

Sunscreen is a chemical agent that denatures light, making the wavelengths incapable of causing damage.

Sunblock is an agent that acts as a physical barrier to prevent sunlight from reaching the surface of the skin.

The key anti-wrinkle concepts are: prevention first, then maintenance, and when all else fails, correction.

screening room

Does your sun protection pass the test? With so many types on the market, it's hard to know which one is best for you.

The difference in texture between cosmetic sunscreens for daily protection and sport sunscreens for outdoor and beach protection is waterproofing. Waterproof lotions have an oil base, which is thicker, heavier and can clog pores. When a product is labelled 'water resistant', it should specify the length of time it will last if you come into contact with water. Labelling varies from country to country and there is no standardization. SPF 15 is considered the minimum you need for it to be effective. Bump that up to SPF 30 if you are playing sports or are on a vacation where you are outdoors more than usual, skiing, swimming or strolling. For spot-prone skin, use an oil-free or non-comedogenic sunscreen. Mineral sunscreens are lighter and wearable under make-up. Zinc oxide is more potent and more expensive, so titanium dioxide is more widely used.

Using a moisturiser that contains a sunscreen can also be misleading. You are unlikely to apply as much of it or use it as often as a regular sunscreen, so it will not be as effective. It may be adequate if you apply it all over your face and neck daily if your sun exposure is limited. It would not be considered enough protection for a day at the beach. What you use on your body is not the same as what you would choose for your face. Most women tend to buy one product for the body and one with a higher SPF for the face. Choose a less pricey formula for your body so

The best sun protectors are a wide-brimmed hat and protective clothing, especially the kind made with cool, light, tightly woven fabrics that keep the sun's rays out. Sunglasses with polarised lenses offer protection for your eyes and from crow's feet.

you'll use more of it. It is critical that you like the fragrance and texture to ensure that you use it daily.

Even if a foundation contains a sunscreen, facial movements throughout the day remove some of it from your face, decreasing its effectiveness. Foundations, concealers, moisturisers, eye creams and lipsticks that offer UVA and UVB protection may be sufficient for normal daily activities. Sebum is produced during the day, thus separating the foundation from the skin's surface. Normal to dry skin types will find it develops at a slower rate. When you are outside, your foundation will only protect you for about 2 hours. After that, either reapply foundation or use a sunscreen over it for continued protection.

In terms of skin cancer prevention, sunscreens alone are imperfect. Studies have shown that people often have the mistaken notion that the higher the SPF, the longer they can stay in the sun, which increases skin exposure. A fair blonde vacationing in the Caribbean generally needs more protection than an olive-skinned brunette walking down the high street in March. The key is that whatever your sunscreen of choice, you must use enough of it and use it regularly. Dermatologists recommend using 1fl oz of lotion per application for one person's whole body.

Don't forget to cover the most burn-prone areas: your lips, eyelids, back of neck, tip of nose, forehead, chest, shoulders and ears.

skin sins

skin sins

If you want to defy ageing, stop smoking and drink less alcohol. Nothing ages skin faster and dehydrates your pores mores than a cigarette and a glass of wine.

You can ALWAYS tell a smoker by her skin. It has a grey or sallow cast, feels dry and is usually lined prematurely, especially around the mouth and eyes. Even if you only have a few cigarettes a day, expect the telltale wrinkles around the mouth and eyes to appear in your 30s.

Scientists have an explanation for what makes smokers look old before their time. Tobacco has been found to activate the genes responsible for the skin enzyme that breaks down collagen, the protein that maintains elasticity in the skin. When this starts to disintegrate, the skin begins to sag and wrinkle. Too much of the enzyme increases the ageing effect of the sun's rays, which also raises the concentration of the enzyme.

Smokers are more prone to getting wrinkles and their skin tends to have a greyish pallor. Smoking causes a flood of free radicals to form in the body, which speeds up the ageing process. Research suggests that smokers have lower levels of vitamin C in their blood than nonsmokers, and that their daily loss of vitamin C is about 35 mg a day greater than nonsmokers'. Women who smoke need to consume at least 110 mg a day of vitamin C to compensate for this loss.

The combination of smoking and sunlight is positively deadly. Plus the nicotine stains on your teeth and fingers are far from glamorous. The

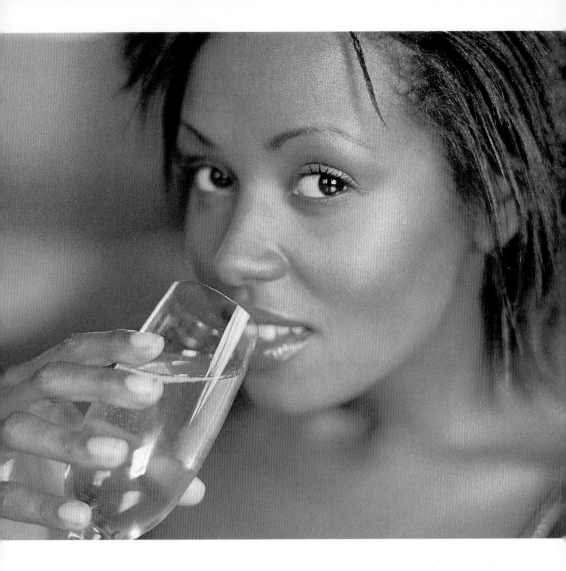

best beauty treatment, and the cheapest, is to QUIT SMOKING.

Steer clear of over-indulging on skin-aggravating alcohol. Aside from hangovers, alcohol can wreak havoc on your skin and give you a puffy face, red and irritated eyes and a washed-out complexion. Alcohol is a diuretic and causes blood vessels to dilate and the skin to lose moisture, resulting in dehydration, sagging and a loss of resiliency. To help your skin stay wrinkle-free, keep cocktails to a minimum.

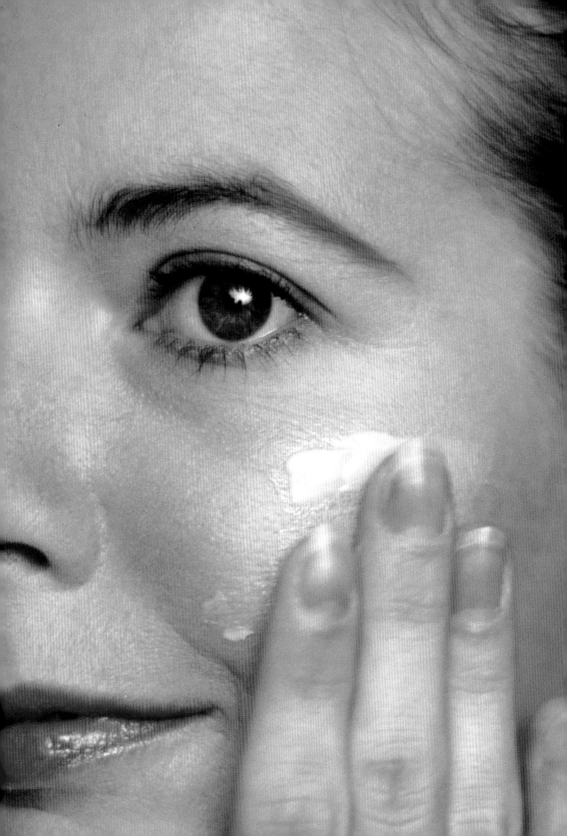

SMOOTHING THEM

SMOOTHING THEM

Wrinkle creams may provide important substances, like vitamins and anitoxidants, but it is never enough to ensure optimum skin nutrition. Some nutrients and metabolites should come from food sources. Others are produced by a healthy well-nourished body. No topical product can replace that. The trick is to look for high concentrations of active ingredients in stable enough forms to be applied topically. Retinoic acid, L-ascorbic acid and alpha hydroxy acids have been the mainstays, but that's just the beginning. While they tackle skin ageing in scientifically different ways, they work synergistically when used together.

Currently there are several clinically-proven active ingredients used in skin rejuvenation, plus a plethora of antioxidants and a vast array of ingredients that play a supporting role. Vitamin A, glycolic acid, N-6 Furfuryladenine, copper peptides, dimethylaminoethanol (DMAE), L-ascorbic acid and alpha lipoic acid are the star performers.

Exfoliation means stripping away the old to bring in the new. On the skin this translates as radiance, vitality and clarity. As cells clump together, you need to jump-start the natural process of sloughing off. There are many modern tools for exfoliation, from sponges, loofahs, flannels and wipes, to peeling agents that penetrate the skin and lasers that strip away the most superficial layers.

beauty boosters

If you're approaching 30, add a few 'active' products to your skin care programme to make sure you reap the benefits of today's advanced technologies.

The term 'active' describes a product containing an ingredient that works beneath the skin's surface, producing visible changes. The active substance should appear in the first 3–5 ingredients on the list. For an ingredient to work, it has to be protected from air and light, reach the target tissue in an active form, be delivered in a high enough concentration to be effective and be used on a regular basis.

Anti-ageing skin care formulations fall into three classifications: over-the-counter (cosmetics); non-prescription (cosmeceuticals); prescription (drugs). Cosmeceuticals include bioactives that have anti-ageing, moisturizing, firming and skin lightening effects. The cosmeceutical category is considered the most scientifically reliable and potent because the products generally contain the highest concentrations of active ingredients.

Beauty and the lab

The key in this age of product overload is to read labels. It's hard to keep up, especially when some ingredients go by more than one name. By law, the first ingredient listed on the label should have the highest concentration in the formula, but every ingredient is listed, even when there are only trace amounts of it in the product.

Skin vitamins

Kinetin (N-6 Furfuryladenine: A naturally occurring growth hormone found in plant and animal DNA with antioxidant and anti-ageing properties.

Copper peptides: Known to aid in the healing of wounds.

Polypeptides: Chains of amino acids linked by peptide bonds.

Vitamin E: Topical natural vitamin E, called d-alpha-tocopherol, reduces sunburn cell production, chronic UV-induced damage.

Alpha Lipoic acid: A super-potent fat and water-soluble antioxidant, which helps reduce UV light-induced inflammation within the skin.

L-ascorbic acid: A form of vitamin C, a water-soluble antioxidant, known for its ability to destroy free radicals.

Dimethylaminoethanol (DMAE): Functions as a cell membrane stabiliser to produce a firming effect.

Niacin: A component of the B vitamin complex with many deriviatives.

Coenzyme Q10: Called ubiquinone, a naturally occurring antioxidant that is present in skin.

Growth Factors: Compounds that act as chemical messengers between cells – turning on and off a variety of cellular activities.

Grapeseed Extract: Contains powerful antioxidants known as oligomeric proanthocyandins (OPCs) or procyanidins.

Vitamin K: Used to lessen redness and reduce the appearance of broken capillaries and bruising.

acid test

AHAs are a group of acids, from fruits and other natural substances, that speed cell turnover and improve texture, reduce fine lines and even out skin tone.

AHAs are key to unclogging embedded cellular debris from pores and shedding the outermost layer of dead skin. They work by consistently peeling away dead and thickened areas of the skin, in essence thinning the build-up. If you stop using AHAs, your skin's turnover rate will gradually become more sluggish. With continued use, AHAs improve a wide range of skin conditions including wrinkles, acne, blotches, and brown spots. Other benefits include their moisturising, oil reduction, and pore-cleansing abilities, as well as bleaching properties for lightening discolouration.

Over-the-counter AHA strengths vary from 4–15 per cent, but are often neutralised to a degree that they are not very effective – 8 per cent is considered the baseline level needed to see results. Sensitive skin types may only be able to tolerate the mildest, like polyhydroxy acids. Glycolic acid is considered to be the most effective AHA for skin rejuvenation because it helps draw other treatments deeper into the skin. At a low pH, it can also aid in stimulating collagen production within the dermis. As the skin becomes conditioned to AHAs, stronger concentrations can be used.

When trying any new product, use it regularly for at least a month before evaluating its

WARNING: Avoid layering acid on acid. Some skin types may only be able to tolerate low potency formulas every other day.

Natural exfoliants

Glycolic acid: Most common AHA, derived from sugarcane or made from synthetic ingredients. Because it is a small molecule, it penetrates the skin easily.
Malic acid: Derived from apples and white grapes.
Tartaric acid: A type of glycolic acid that results from the fermentation process used in making wine.
Uses: Exfoliation, reducing surface oils, unclogging blackheads, smoothing fine lines.

Beta hydroxy acid: Also referred to as salicylic acid. It does not penetrate as deeply into the dermis as glycolic acid, so it is less irritating.
Uses: Exfoliation of epidermis, prevention of clogged pores.

Citric acid: Derived from citrus fruits. Acts as an antioxidant on the skin.
Uses: May stimulate collagen production, has mild bleaching properties.

Lactic acid: Comes from sour milk. Works as an exfoliator and to hold water in the skin as a component of the skin's natural moisturising mechanism.
Uses: Softening thick, rough skin, moisturising.

Polyhydroxy acids: Considered one of the mildest formulations because they are larger molecules so are limited in the way they can penetrate the skin.
Uses: Softening thick, rough skin, moisturising.

effectiveness. Your skin fluctuates with your monthly cycle. In order to determine whether a product is working, you need to use it during each phase of that cycle. Don't try more than one new product at a time, as it will be hard to tell how your skin responds to any of them. Buy products with adequate labelling: for example, a list of ingredients and the name and address of the manufacturer or distributor. Stop using a product immediately if you experience any adverse reactions, including stinging, redness, itching, burning or increased sun sensitivity.

gimme an 'A'

When you hit 30, skin can begin to look dull. Vitamin A is still the mother of all anti-ageing treatments. It is essential for normal skin development, increases skin elasticity and dermal thickening, and reverses photoageing.

Tretinoin isn't the only form of topical vitamin A anymore. Other forms include retinyl palmitate, retinol and tazarotene, and more are on their way. Renova (Retinova) and Avage (Tazarotene) are both approved by the US FDA to treat ageing skin.

Tretinoin: A pure form of vitamin A, it can reduce fine lines, fade age spots, clear pimples and control rosacea. Originally prescribed for acne, Retin-A (whose active ingredient is tretinoin) has been found to do much more. It exfoliates the surface of the skin, unblocking clogged pores and forces the cells below to regenerate more quickly. It acts as a peeling agent that helps the skin renew itself more rapidly, treating and preventing photoageing. The result is smoother skin thanks to the increase of collagen and elastin fibres. To see visible improvement, you have to use it for at least a month and the improvement will last only as long as it is used. It also makes the skin more sun-sensitive, so sun protection and avoiding sunlamps is vital. It does have the potential to irritate, so if you have a reaction to it, try skipping a day, using it every 2 days or just applying it to wrinkle-prone areas like crow's-feet, forehead lines and around the lips. You can also experiment with 'short contact therapy', i.e. using a thin coat and washing it off after 10 minutes, so penetration is limited. Start with a low concentration and work your way up until you reach the highest concentration that your skin can tolerate and use it on a regular basis. Tretinoin is used in concentrations of 0.025, 0.05 and 0.01 per cent and microencapsulated forms.

Tretinoin emollient cream: This prescription cream is basically Retin-A in a moisturising base that is ideally suited to dry, ageing skin. It should be applied exactly as prescribed, once a day at bedtime. Do not apply more or use it more often. Your wrinkles will not disappear any faster and skin may be irritated. Retinova may be too rich if your skin is oily or acne-prone. Tretinoin emollient cream is available in concentrations of 0.02 or 0.05 per cent.

Retinol: An over-the-counter vitamin A derivative that stimulates cell division and reduces fine lines over time. Small amounts of retinol are converted by the skin to retinoic acid, the main ingredient in Retin-A. Retinols are not as effective and you won't see results as quickly. Over-the-counter formulas contain as little as 0.1 per cent up to a maximum 5 per cent.

Good medicine

Instructions for use:
- Before applying the cream, wash your face with mild soap.
- Pat it dry and wait then 20–30 minutes before applying the cream.
- Use a pea-size amount to cover the face.
- Wash your hands after applying it.
- Daily use of an SPF 15 is essential.

Possible side effects:
Flaking, dryness, stinging, burning, redness, irritation.

wrinkle relief

wrinkle relief

Prior to the advent of cosmeceuticals, we had two basic choices for looking more youthful: make-up or surgery. Now, when your skin seems to be heading south, before you book a date with a scalpel, check your bathroom cabinet.

The basis of all effective anti-ageing skin care should be broad spectrum sunscreen in the morning and a treatment product like retinoid at night. Every regime can be altered in special situations as needed. Take into account your age, lifestyle, skin type and what you are hoping to achieve from your skin care. Moisturising products are not going to turn back the clock alone. Before you invest in a pricey regime, do your homework.

Determine your skin type: Are you mostly oily, dry, normal, sensitive or combination? Do a self-test to make sure: wash your face, wait 30 minutes and then put a single piece of tissue paper against your forehead, nose, chin and cheeks. Oily areas will leave a residue on the tissue paper.

Identify your complexion:
I. Very fair skin – never tans, always burns
II. Light skin – may tan, but usually burns
III. Light to medium complexion – sometimes tans, sometimes burns
IV. Medium complexion – usually tans, rarely burns
V. Dark complexion – never burns
VI. Black complexion – never burns

Prioritise your concerns: Do you want preventative maintenance to avoid premature ageing? Do you have a skin problem, such as acne, melasma or rosacea? Are large pores, sun damage, wrinkles or fine lines your primary concern? Do you have eye puffiness or under eye bags? List all that apply to you.

Assess your lifestyle: Are you a smoker? Do you spend a lot of time in the sun? Do you eat a well-balanced diet and get enough exercise? All these factors will affect how you should care for your skin.

Product usage

Be careful about layering products, which can result in irritation or product interaction that may negate their effects and sensitise your skin. Avoid using the same ingredient or competing ingredients in too many products at the same time. Separate acidic products by using one in the AM and one in the PM instead.

Skin care budgeting

Price is not an indicator of efficacy. Sticking to your beauty budget is all about prioritising, but an overly frugal approach may sabotage your beauty regime. Don't cut corners where it counts. Cheaper products can sometimes mean sacrificing the key ingredients you skin craves. Less expensive formulas often contain more water and so you need more of it to get the job done. High quality products may be extra concentrated, so a little bit goes a long way.

antioxidants

In ageing skin cells, naturally occuring antioxidants are in short supply. Many compounds used in anti-ageing skin care have antioxidant properties to replace those that diminish with age.

A potent skin rejuvenation programme should incorporate alpha hydroxy acids (AHAs) with one fibroblast-stimulating antioxidant: GHK copper peptides, L-ascorbic acid or Alpha lipoic acid (ALA). Together these ingredients have the ability to repair and protect the skin, and prevent further damage.

While there are many new agents on the horizon for skin rejuvenation, vitamin A was the first antioxidant to be widely used in skin care. Vitamin C is technically an AHA (citric acid) but is additionally a potent antioxidant. It has been used effectively to stimulate collagen repair, thus diminishing some of the effects of photoageing. Topical natural vitamin E can ease chronic UV-induced damage and soothe dry, rough skin. When vitamin E is combined with vitamin C, both vitamins create a highly protective barrier against sun damage.

Alpha lipoic acid (ALA) is a super-potent fat- and water-soluble antioxidant; it is different from most other antioxidants, which are either one or the other. ALA can penetrate skin cells easily through the lipid rich cell membrane and continue to be effective once inside the cell due to its water solubility. ALA has also been shown to have a protective effect on vitamins C and e, thereby boosting naturally occuring antioxidants within the cell.

First recognised for their ability to enhance wound healing, copper peptides are known to improve skin strength, thicken the dermis and increase blood vessel formation and oxygenation within the skin. One of its main

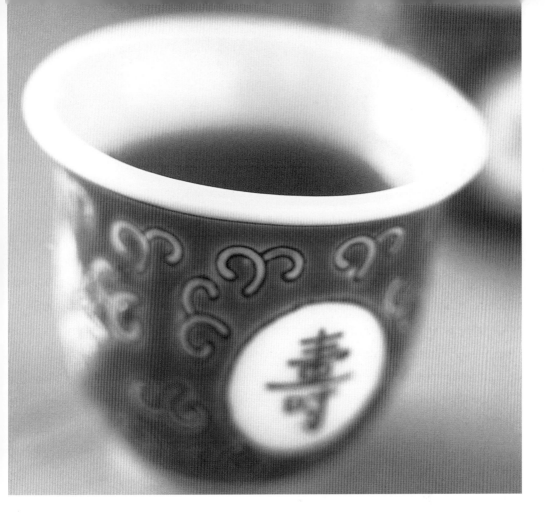

advantages is that it is non-irritating and relatively inexpensive compared to other antioxidant creams. Copper peptide formulas are ideal for sensitive skin, rosacea or eczema or anyone looking for a gentle skin rejuvenation option.

Grapeseed extract contains powerful antioxidants known as oligomeric proanthocyanidins (OPCs) or procyanidins. Pyconogenol from pinebark extract and constituents of wine, cranberries, green and black teas, blackcurrants, onions and hawthorn are similar in their active ingredients and medicinal uses. Coenzyme Q10, called ubiquinone, is a naturally occuring antioxidant that is present in skin. Topical application of Coenzyme Q10 has been shown to prevent peroxidation of cell membrane lipids.

future skin

Skin care technology sounds like a biochemistry lesson. Many of the newer products have taken their lead from the science behind wound healing.

There is no perfect skin rejuvenation product and no magical therapy that does it all. Each ingredient is derived from a different source, is active in a different way and produces different results than the next. One is also not necessarily better than the other. However, by incorporating several key ingredients together into a skin care routine, the skin receives improved synergistic benefits than by using one over the other. Some ingredients have a place as a stand alone product or they might be used as part of a multi-step approach. For example, a glycolic peel followed by the application of topical growth factor may increase the penetration of the growth factors, which may reduce inflammation and speed healing.

Growth factors

This new category of compounds being used to treat ageing skin is extracted from cultured epidermal cells, placental cells, human foreskin and even plants, growth factors are compounds that act as chemical messengers between cells – turning on and off a variety of cellular activities. Growth factors are a group of proteins that perform a vast array of functions in human growth and development. Each member of the growth factor family binds to a unique receptor and they work alone and in concert to regulate specific types of cells and tissues. They contain a number of active compounds, some of which are important in collagen synthesis. Common Human Growth Factors include Transforming Growth Factor-beta (TGF-beta), Vascular Endothelial Growth Factor (VEGF), Platelet-derived Growth Factor (PDGF) and Keratinocyte Growth Factor.

Spin traps

Compounds called spin traps are at the cutting edge of cosmeceutical advancements. Known for their ability to bind free radical, spin traps have been used primarily in the lab setting in the past but are now being looked at as therapeutic agents. Spin traps have antioxidant and anti-inflammatory properties, and have been shown to be beneficial in treating inflammatory conditions like rosacea and sunburn.

Expert advice: Look at the science behind the claims. They should have some clinical evidence to back them up. Don't accept every wrinkle cure at face value. It is often difficult to determine whether claims about the action or efficacy of cosmeceuticals are valid. Just because a product has a logical mechanism of action doesn't mean that it will necessarily reduce wrinkles. What works well in the lab may not be feasible in the real world because of packaging issues, shelf life, loss of potency over time, instability and exposure to the environment. Many products make the skin feel better and that, in turn, makes women feel that they are really changing their skin. If you go from using nothing on your skin, or taking a casual attitude towards skin care, you are going to be shocked to see the difference in your skin when you get going on a proper regime that has some thought behind it.

peel me a grape

Superficial peels basically accomplish three key things: exfoliation, moisturisation and thickening the dermis. Any acid can be made to penetrate the skin lightly or deeply.

Peels vary according to their active ingredients, strength, how long the solution remains on the skin and the pH. Diverse peeling agents penetrate to different levels and, consequently, produce varying results. They all involve applying a chemical solution to remove damaged outer layers so that newer layers can replace the old ones. Peels can reduce wrinkles and fine lines around the eyes and mouth, sun spots, hyperpigmentation, melasma, scarring, some types of acne and actinic keratoses or precancerous lesions. The deeper a peel penetrates, the more visible results you can achieve, but the lengthier the recovery period. Most peels can be performed on the face, neck, chest, hands, arms and legs.

A peel treatment begins with cleansing the skin and removing all traces of grease with alcohol or acetone. The face is then rinsed with water and blown-dry with a small fan. A solution is applied using a sponge, cotton pad, cotton swab or brush to the areas evenly. A grey-white film, referred to as 'frost', develops by the end of the application. The peeling solution is left on for a few minutes and then neutralised with water.

The most commonly performed peels use mild solutions of beta hydroxy acid, glycolic acid, lactic acid and salicylic acid, to lightly peel the skin. They are typically done in a series to maintain results over time and the process usually takes 10–20 minutes. Superficial peels are usually combined with an at home skin care regimen for best results. The solution used will typically be adjusted for each treatment session based on your skin's response.

Medium Peels like Jessner's Solution and Trichloroacetic Acid (TCA) are used to correct pigment problems, superficial blemishes, moderate sun damage, fine lines and weathered skin. TCA peels are performed in a doctors office. Anesthesia is usually not necessary. You may feel a warm or burning sensation which is followed by some stinging.

Deeper Peels with Phenol and croton oil are usually a one off procedure. They can produce more dramatic, long-term results on wrinkles, brown spots, scarring and pre-cancerous growths. Because these permanently lighten skin, they are not recommended for darker skin tones and require that sunscreen be used afterwards. A deep full-face peel requires intravenous sedation and takes one or two hours, while a deep peel to a smaller area on the face, such as the upper lip, may take only 15 minutes.

Deeper peels give better results, but look worse afterwards and take longer to heal. With lighter peels, you need more treatments. Deeper peels carry a greater risk of skin bleaching (hypo-pigmentation), skin discolouration (hyper-pigmentation), a demarcation line or scarring.

WARNING: DO NOT have any peel if you are taking RoAccutane or if you have herpes simplex or other open lesions. If you have a history of cold sores, ask your doctor for an antiviral before having a peel or laser treatment around the mouth.

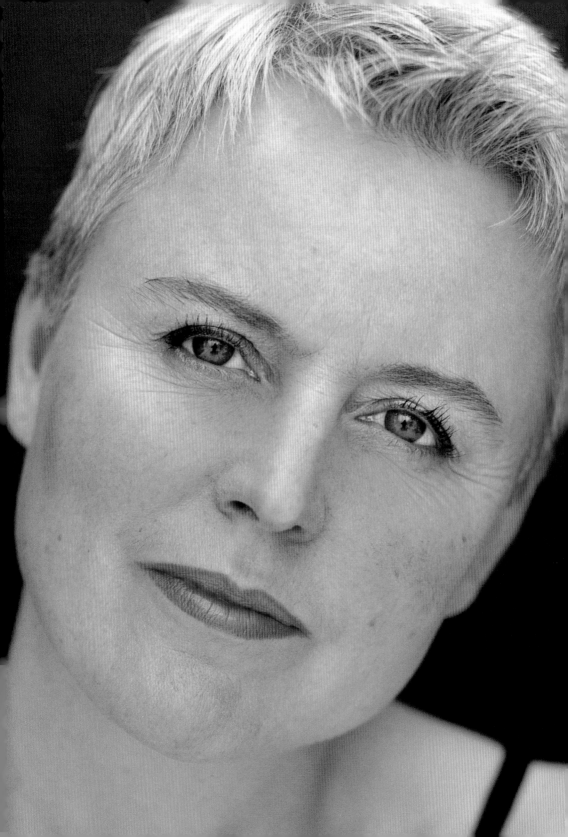

ZAPPING
THEM

ZAPPING THEM

Topical skin-care products only do so much to improve the appearance of the skin. If you want to see more dramatic improvements, you have to look to deeper remedies, the kind of treatments performed by cosmetic surgeons, dermatologists, nurses and medical aestheticians. There is a wide choice of facial rejuvenation techniques, making it possible to tailor therapies to your exact needs. Resurfacing methods can remove the top layers of the skin, revealing unblemished, unlined skin below.

Lasers can treat acne scarring, acne lesions, age spots, birthmarks, hair removal, hemangiomas, red birthmarks, hyperpigmentation, moles, port wine stains, psoriasis, raised scars, repigmentation, skin cancers, thread veins, sun damage, tattoo removal, varicose veins and wrinkles. They can also be used to repigment skin that has been whitened or scars that appear lighter than your normal skin colour. Unlike the deeper lasers, non-ablative lasers offer less invasive treatment that improves skin texture and tone by stimulating new collagen in the skin to smooth it out from underneath. These treatments do not destroy outer tissue as they work their way down to stimulate collagen growth in the dermis. Each device delivers controlled energy to the skin in slightly different ways, but the process is gradual and the softening of wrinkles occurs over time as the rejuvenated fibres reach the skin surface. The newest light sources are being used for skin contraction to tighten the skin for a non-surgical lifting effect.

resurfacing
rules

resurfacing rules

Laser resurfacing can remove wrinkles and red veins, lighten discolourations and age spots, and smooth scars, as well as stimulate fibroblasts to increase collagen production.

A laser is a high-energy beam of light that selectively directs its energy into tissue. It works like a scalpel that allows the doctor greater control and finesse. It applies the principles of radiation physics to narrowly segregate light of a selected wavelength and 'pump' the light radiation to high intensity. The beams are targeted to a specific spot and are varied in intensity and in the duration of emitted pulses depending on their mission. Lasers and light sources are the modern way to pulverize wrinkles and extract redness from the skin. They have virtually left many older techniques in the dust.

Resurfacing with a laser should only be performed by a medical doctor. It can be done under local anaesthetic with or without intravenous sedation, or anaesthetic cream or spray can be used for more superficial procedures. Depending on the extent of the treatment, it can take anywhere from a few minutes to more than an hour. The laser is passed over parts of the face, neck, chest or hands, and evaporates the surface layers of the targeted areas of skin. A new layer of pink skin is revealed. Generally, the more passes with the laser and the deeper the setting, the more extensive the treatment and longer the recovery.

The newest lasers penetrate to the layers beneath to boost collagen production, giving skin a plumper, tighter appearance. Treatments improve skin texture and tone by stimulating new collagen in the skin to smooth it out from underneath the surface. These treatments do not destroy outer tissue as they stimulate collagen growth in the dermis, so they are safe to use on most skin types. The process is gradual and the softening of wrinkles occurs over time. You will need multiple treatment sessions in order to see results. No pain, no gain. Don't expect to be wrinkle-free at the end of one course. The advantage is zero recovery time so you won't be red for months.

The darker the skin colour, the more risk of lightening, darkening, or scarring from resurfacing treatments. If you have freckles on parts of your face, deeper laser resurfacing performed on one regional area like around the mouth, the lower eyelid area, or the forehead, instead of the full face, may leave you with an uneven appearance. Although the lighter lasers are not able to eradicate wrinkles and brown spots as well, they are more appealing to women who are unwilling or unable to put up with a long recovery. Non-ablative techniques are also good for anyone who can't commit to staying out of the sun. For extensive sun damage, higher wavelengths may be required.

New lasers are being used to treat stretch marks, whitened scars, acne scars, burns and resurfaced skin to restore pigment that has been lost. These light-based therapies improve the appearance of lightened scars by restoring pigment. Multiple treatments may be needed and repigmentation can last for several years depending on the extent of the hyperpigementation.

BEAUTY BYTE:
For more about anti-wrinkle lasers, visit www.aslms.org and www.asds-net.org.

high beams

high beams

Ablative laser resurfacing is not a casual undertaking. Doctors love the effects of the carbon dioxide laser, but the downside is prolonged healing and redness.

Everyone knows someone who turned scarlet after a laser treatment and seemed to stay like that forever, making ablative lasers almost a thing of the past as dermabrasion was before the advent of lasers. Deeper lasers are being used more superficially so that you can look good after a week and the pinkness fades quickly. These treatments are good for more severe sun damage, wrinkles and deep acne scarring, but they are slowly being replaced by less invasive models.

Carbon Dioxide – The Carbon Dioxide laser is considered the workhorse of laser devices. The treatment can reach the deeper wrinkles because it heats the tissues more intensely. This is a more serious treatment with a longer recovery period. When energy is delivered into the skin over a certain temperature, superficial tissues are vaporized and ablated or destroyed. CO2 is still considered the original skin resurfacing laser because of its ability to cause skin shrinkage and its dramatic results on deeper wrinkles. However, in some circles, the mere mention of the word 'laser' conjures up fears of a red, swollen, crusty face.

Erbiym:YAG – Erbium:YAG technology has gained acceptance as the second cousin to Cardon Dioxide, but without some of the side effects.

The milder Erbium:YAG works well on fine lines and wrinkles, mild sun damage and scars. These lasers target the skin itself and the wavelengths are absorbed by water. Since most of our cells are predominantly water, these wavelengths are absorbed by the first cells they touch. The heat effects of the laser are scattered so that thin layers of tissue can be removed with precision while minimizing damage to the surrounding skin. Long pulse Erbium:YAG lasers deliver results that fall somewhere between the CO2 and the Erbium:YAG. If needed, you can repeat the treatment in the future. The treatment is like a medium depth peel and works best for mild to moderate skin damage.

Electrosurgical Resurfacing – Electrosurgical resurfacing, also called 'cold ablation' or coblation, uses a micro-electrical radio frequency to deliver a pulse of energy instead of heat to the surface of the skin to improve moderate damage. It seals blood vessels as it removes tissue and promotes skin tightening as a laser would, but by a dramatically cooler process. Electrosurgical resurfacing is applicable to most skin types and colours, without loss of skin pigmentaton. The swelling and redness usually clears in 2–4 weeks. It can be used to improve superficial to moderate skin damage and is generally a less expensive alternative with slightly faster healing than some lasers, but the benefits to lines and wrinkles may not last as long.

BEAUTY BYTES:

For more info on lasers, log on to

www.skinandhealth.com

laser toning

laser toning

Lunchtime treatments with no downtime or redness are definitely what women want, even though the results will not be as dramatic. Lasers and light sources can accomplish this goal.

Non-ablative lasers and light sources work on the deeper layers of the skin without removing the top layer. These treatments do not burn or destroy outer tissue as they work their way down to stimulate new collagen growth in the dermis. Each device delivers controlled energy to the skin in slightly different ways. The process is gradual and the softening of wrinkles occurs over time as the rejuvenated skin fibres reach the surface. All systems require treatments to be repeated every 4–6 weeks and a minimum of 3 treatments are needed. Most common types are infrared lasers, visible light lasers and broadband light sources.

Since these lasers often have a long wavelength, they are safe for a variety of skin types. There may be some discomfort similar to a rubber band snapping against the skin. Topical anaesthetic may be used to numb the skin. These systems are ideal for maintenance after more aggressive or deeper resurfacing, or as part of a maintenance program in combination with skin care, peels or microdermabrasion. Most people see some improvement in 30 days and may continue to see improvements for up to 90 days. The newly formed collagen will then age at a normal rate and you can repeat the procedure as needed. They can be used to treat the face, neck, chest, hands and legs.

TOP TIP:

Don't get too hung up on the names of these systems because they change so frequently.

Intense Pulsed Light Sources These multi-purpose systems work by creating a wound in the small blood vessels in the dermis that causes collagen and blood vessels under the top layer to constrict. Light energy is delivered through the skin to remove redness, pigment, reduce pore size, minimise fine lines and for hair removal. After a few treatments, your skin will have more even and smooth tone. If you have rosacea and facial flushing, you can expect to see a reduction in redness after each treatment. IPLs work for fine lines particularly around the eyes and mouth, brown spots, thread veins, large pores and chronic facial redness.

Radiofrequency Waves Devices utilising radiofrequency waves are being used to tighten loose skin on the neck, brows and other face and body areas. They work by delivering deep intense heat into the skin without injury to the epidermis. The system is comprised of a radio frequency (RF) generator; a controlled modular cooling system that houses a cryogen canister and related cooling control components; and a hand-held treatment tip that couples both the cryogen cooling and the RF heating device to the area. One or more treatments may be needed, and some anaesthetic is necessary. This technology is being touted as a non-surgical lift.

LED Technology Unlike laser technology that relies on high-powered coherent light to create heat energy, LED photomodulation triggers the body to convert light energy into cell energy without damaging the tissues with heat. Treatment involves sitting in front of a panel of low level light-emitting diodes (LEDs).

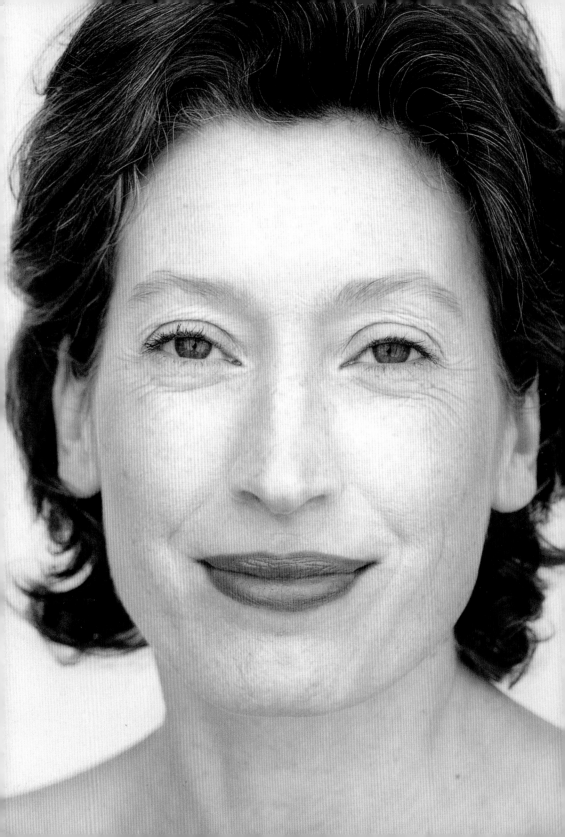

NEEDLE POINTS

There comes a point in every woman's life when all the creams, peels and lasers together aren't enough to plump up lines, creases and canyons. That's the time to look to wrinkle fillers, which are another method to add to your maintenance program. All of the minimally invasive treatments described in this book complement each other. Think of wrinkle remedies like a menu in a Chinese restaurant. Take a bit from each column to put together your perfect rejuvenation menu, and add to it as the lines get deeper. The best method is an integrated approach that may begin with one or a combination of parasurgical treatments until you are ready (or willing) to go under the knife.

Botulinum toxin has become the cornerstone of any anti-ageing programme for the face. No other single product has revolutionised cosmetic medicine so much in such a relatively short time. BOTOX® is not a filler like bovine collagen or fat. It relaxes muscles to make the lines disappear and can slow down the formation of new lines. Most fillers temporarily plump up creases but don't prevent them from getting deeper or stop new ones from forming. Fillers are used to add volume to the face, which BOTOX® cannot do. Fillers work better in deep creases, cheeks and lips. These treatments are not mutually exclusive, but rather complimentary. It also gives the best value for money.

beauty of Botox

Botox has proved to be a little poison with unlimited health and beauty potential. A few precious drops can manage everything from frown lines, worry lines, upper lip creases, and neck cords, to excessive sweating and migraines.

After getting over the idea of having a toxin injected into their faces, most women get hooked. Just one treatment brings a noticeable improvement and softening of facial lines. There is literally no age that is too soon to start, and women in their late 20s and 30s are into botulinum toxin in a big way as part of an early battle against ageing. Unlike fillers that plump up creases, Botox slows down the formation of new facial lines and smooths the lines already there.

New uses are discovered constantly, as doctors are becoming more experimental with its potent effects. For example, it is now commonly used to rejuvenate the upper face, mid face, lower face and neck.

Where it works

Vertical lines between the brows

Lines at the bridge of the nose

Crow's-feet or squint lines

Horizontal forehead lines

Lifting the droopy nasal tip

Under eyelid creases, muscle rolls

Décolleté lines, neck bands

Chin creases and dimples

Drooping corners of the mouth

Upper and lower lip lines

How Botox works

The toxin acts on the junctions between nerves and muscles, preventing the release of a chemical messenger, acetylcholine, from the nerve endings. Tiny amounts are injected into a specific facial muscle so only the targeted impulse of that muscle is blocked, immobilising the underlying cause of the unwanted lines – muscle contractions – and prevent lines and wrinkles. Since the muscle can no longer make the offending facial expression, the lines gradually smooth out from disuse and new creases are prevented from forming. Untreated muscles are not affected, so a natural look and expressions are maintained. Some areas are less suited to this procedure because the muscles are needed for expression and important functions like eating, kissing and opening the eyes. The goal is a softening of dynamic facial lines that won't necessarily betray your wrinkle-reducing secret. There are various strains of Botulinum toxin. Type A is the most potent and commonly used.

Botulinum toxin type A: Pioneered by an ophthalmologist in 1987, its wide range of cosmetic uses has made it a mainstay in the cosmetic surgeon's arsenal of weapons for mass destruction of facial wrinkles. It received approval for cosmetic use in the US in 2002 and is available under the trade name Botox Cosmetic (Allergan) and Dysport (Ipsen Ltd).

Botulinum toxin type B: Marketed under the name MYOBLOC in the US and NeuroBloc in the EC (Elan Pharmaceuticals) it is approved for use in the treatment of cervical dystonia, a neurological disorder, and not yet approved for cosmetic uses. This form comes as a premade liquid that does not require a diluting agent, and is typically preserved in normal saline. Compared with Type A, it has a longer shelf life of up to 2 years and works slightly faster but it can be more painful when injected.

frozen assets

frozen assets

- Have your first treatment with someone who comes highly recommended and has a lot of experience, so that you will know what is acceptable.

- Start small with one area, typically the lines between the brows or crow's-feet. Once you see the results, you can have more areas worked on at your next treatment.

- If you are squeamish about needles, ask your doctor for a topical anaesthetic cream or gel.

- To relieve the discomfort of the injections, apply an ice pack before and after treatment.

- If your treatment didn't work, you may have been given an overly diluted solution and need more, or it could have been injected into the wrong spot. It is exceedingly rare to be resistant to it.

- Take along a concealer to cover needle marks or tiny bruises right after treatment. Have your Botox treatment at least a week before any big social event.

- Don't have a treatment without having eaten to avoid getting lightheaded.

- Botulinum toxin isn't the answer for all your wrinkles. It doesn't work as well on lines that are not entirely caused by muscle activity, like the nasal labial folds that are formed by a combination of muscle action and the weight of sagging skin.

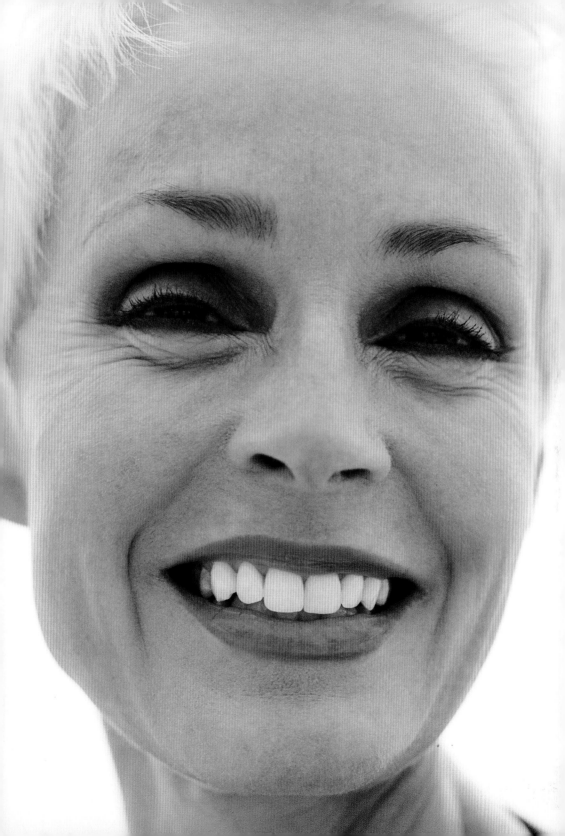

Botox budgeting

Botox budgeting

Botulinum toxin takes effect 2–7 days after treatment. The improvement generally lasts for 3–6 months, before the effect gradually fades and muscle action returns.

Doctors set their fees by the area, by the treatment, or based on how much material they inject. Each area to be treated is considered a zone; for example, the crow's-feet on both sides of your face would be considered one zone; horizontal forehead lines constitute another zone; the frown lines between your eyebrows would be another zone. Each zone is usually priced separately, but most doctors discount the fee for the second and third areas. The most common combination of areas to have done in one go is: between the eyebrows, the forehead, and the crow's-feet. If you decide to do a little more for this line or that, because he is there already, don't be surprised to be charged an additional amount. Ask ahead of time what the fee will be for your treatment so you are prepared.

A single treatment will normally be sustained for up to 4 months, with some variation. In areas where there are two sides to be injected, as in the forehead or crow's-feet, the toxin may fade unevenly and the lines on one side return more than the lines on the other. When you begin to notice a gradual fading of its effects, you should have your next treatment. Don't wait until all of it has worn off – keep up with your treatments. When you are able to contract your facial muscles, go back for a touch-up. If you stay on top of it, you will look consistently unlined all the time. If you wait 6 months between treatments, until all or most of it has worn off, it will be a telltale sign that you are a Botox user. Basically, you can expect to have a treatment 3–4 times a year. Beware of discounted Botox – you may be paying less because you are getting less. Some doctors overdilute the solution or keep it around for too long, causing it to lose its potency. The result is that your wrinkles won't stay frozen as well or for as long. Instead of getting a good result for 4 months, it may only last for 2, and there goes your savings!

Some people have more active muscles that require more injections, like men, and require more intense and more frequent treatments. In some cases, the more treatments you have, the longer it will last between treatments, but that is not true for everyone.

The real deal

Very little can go wrong with botulinum toxin, and the good news is that if it does, it is temporary. The only complications are an occasional eyelid droop, an asymmetry, or a crooked mouth. Side effects are rarely serious and always temporary, and even if you don't like the results, they are guaranteed to go away as it wears off. The problems are about technique, and some doctors are just simply better than others.

You may bruise slightly at the injection site. To avoid bruising, don't take aspirin, anti-inflammatories or vitamin E for a week before. Avoid treatment while you are menstruating, when your body is more sensitive. Some people get a slight headache that can last for a few days. After treatment, you must smile and frown a lot for 2–3 hours and avoid massaging the area, so it stays where it was injected. It is a good idea to go back for a touch-up after 2–3 weeks in case any fine-tuning is needed. If too much is injected or it is placed incorrectly, the toxin can travel to nearby muscles and cause curious expressions or uneven brows.

rejuvenation by the needle

Wrinkle fillers are very versatile. They can be used both as a precursor to a facelift as well as an adjunct and an alternative for the scalpel shy.

As you turn the corner from your 30s to your 40s, one of the first signs of ageing is the loss of the soft, round, cherubic fullness. As you age, you need all the fat you can get in your face, and it's harder to keep it off your body. It's all about proportions. The little fat pad under the chin and pouches along the jawline start to expand. As the natural fullness of your face changes shape, hollows start to show up around the eyelids, the middle of the cheeks and around the mouth. Putting fullness back into hollows and sunken areas softens the changes associated with ageing, and there are many substances to get the job done.

Hyaluronic Acid Gel is the most universally accepted of all wrinkle fillers. There are many brands available, and Restylane/Perlane (QMed) is derived from bacterial fermantation so it is non-animal and therefore considered the most purified. HA is a safe material that is naturally found in the connective tissues of the body, and often the commercial filler of choice.

NewFill (Dermik) is based on a substance called polylactic acid which occurs naturally and has been used in suture material. It stimulates production of the body's own collagen within the line or wrinkle, and can be used in the lips, naso-labial fold, cheeks and scars. Either 2 or 3 treatments are recommended, and it is considered a safe substance.

Your own fat can be taken from one body area and transplanted to plump up lips, cheeks, chins, furrows and hollows, and fill scars. Fat works best as a volume filler for deeper creases and folds, not fine lines. The fat is layered below the skin to create a supportive structure in the face. Donor fat is taken with a small cannula or sterile tube from hips or thighs, processed to remove any blood or serum, and then re-injected into the areas to be filled. When this technique is done in stages, it allows for a gradual improvement over time without a long recovery. Your fat can be kept frozen for up to a year, which enables additional corrections to be made. Fat transfer is also a good complement to cosmetic surgery.

Another process of using your own tissues for filling is called Isolagen™. Your own fibroblasts or collagen producing cells are extracted, reproduced and then injected into folds and crease. As these collagen-forming cells gradually diminish, the skin's support system is weakened and the signs of ageing begin to appear. The treatment starts with a biopsy procedure to take a small 3mm piece of skin tissue from behind your ear which is sent for processing. After about 8 weeks, the cells will be sent back to your doctor's office for your treatments. A series of injections are usually done, spaced about two weeks apart, to correct your wrinkles.

CosmoDerm and CosmoPlast (Inamed) contain human collagen that has been purified from a single cell culture. It contains 0.3 per cent lidocaine to help with pain management. These are injected just below the surface of the skin to fill in superficial lines and wrinkles and to define the border of the lips, and it typically lasts 2–4 months.

long shots

A face-lift doesn't get rid of wrinkles. Lasers don't fill up folds. When wrinkles deepen into folds and creases, they need to be plumped up.

It seems as though anything that can fit into a syringe can be injected into wrinkles. Only medical doctors and registered nurses are licensed to administer injections. Be careful about using an injector whose qualifications you are not sure about or who has very little experience.

Fillers can be broken down into 2 basic categories: resorbable and non-resorbable.

Resorbable fillers: Resorbable fillers are made from natural or synthetic materials that are broken down and resorbed by the body over time. They are temporary and will need to be repeated, typically in 3–9 months on average. If you are not happy with the results, it will eventually disappear. You can have other fillers injected into the same area later on.

Non-resorbable fillers: This class of fillers has synthetic components that don't get broken down by the body. They are considered 'permanent' because the particles cannot be removed or 'semi-permanent' because the particles are suspended in a substance that gets resorbed in 3–6 months, or because the entire material breaks down over time. The term 'permanent' is somewhat misleading. As the ageing process continues, you will need additional treatments down the line.

Wrinkle fillers

Type	Brand Name
Resorbable	
Animal derived	
Bovine collagen	Zyplast, Zyderm
Hyaluronic acid gel	Hylaform, Hylaform Plus, Hylaform Fine
Non-animal derived	
Hyaluronic acid gel	Restylane, Restylane Fine, Perlane, Juvederm, AcHyal, MacDermol
Polylactic acid	NewFill
Human tissue	Derived from human cadaveric tissue from a bank or autologous tissues from your body
Tissue banks	Fascialata – Fascian
	Dermis – Cymetra*, AlloDerm
	Collagen – Cosmoplast™, Cosmoderm™
Autologous cultured fibroblasts	Isolagen Autologistic Tissue Injection
Non-resorbable	
Permanent	
Liquid silicone	Silikon 1000, SilSkin
Semi-permanent	
Bovine collagen PMMA particles	ArteColl, ArteFill
Hyaluronic acid acrylic hydrogel	Dermalive
Calcium Hydroxyl/Apatite	Radiance

This is a partial list, including just the fillers most commonly used in the US. Trade names vary depending on the country or region.

between the lines

Wrinkle fillers are like buses. A new one comes along every 30 minutes. It takes a long time to establish the long-term safety of new formulas.

There are currently over 70 fillers on the market worldwide. Many of these are not tested, have little clinical data supporting their use and are just plain unsafe. The safest fillers are typically temporary treatments that have a long track record and are manufactured by a reputable company. Longer lasting fillers come with possible complications that include lumping, inflammation, granulomas or localised hardening, rash and the migration of microspheres into other areas.

ArteColl® (Rofil) is a semi-permanent filler made of 75 per cent bovine collagen and 25 per cent polymethyl-methacrylate microspheres (PMMA), which are carbon-based polymers. The product is mixed with lidocaine to numb the area to be injected. Over 3 months, the collagen fibres get absorbed, leaving the PMMA, which are too large to be broken down and remain. ArteColl® can be used for acne scars and for filling depressions such as cheeks and folds.

Radiance™ (Bioform) is composed of calcium hydroxyl apatite, which is used in the body for multiple applications including cheek and chin implants. Radiance™ adds volume to the face through mircospheres that are suspended in polysaccharide carriers until they get encapsulated. It can last from 2–4 years.

Liquid silicone is making a comeback in a sterile, purified injectable grade form. It is injected with a micro droplet technique, which has the advantage of causing fewer hard lumps. Not all forms of silicone are created equal and it varies by degree of purity.

filler questions

Questions to ask your doctor

- What is the source of the material?

- Is it natural or synthetic?

- What is the name of the manufacturer and where are they located? (Ask to see a product brochure.)

- How long has the filler been on the market?

- What kinds of clinical studies have been carried out on the filler?

- Is it FDA-approved, or does it have the EC mark?

- How long has the doctor/nurse been using it?

- What are the possible side effects?

- Do I need a skin test before treatment?

- Could I be allergic to the filler?

- What does a reaction look like and how long does it last?

- What can be done if I have a reaction to it?

- What are the risks?

- How many treatments will I need and how often?

- How much will each treatment cost?

- If it doesn't look right, what can be done to remove it?

- Can I still have other fillers later on?

choosing a surgeon

choosing a surgeon

Before any procedure, consult with at least three surgeons to get educated. Check out websites, research credentials and insist on board certification in an appropriate speciality. If you are having surgery done in an outpatient setting, make sure the facility is fully accredited. Find the best doctors possible for whatever procedure you are considering.

General questions to ask before any surgery

- What can I reasonably expect as a final result from this procedure? If appropriate, ask to meet a patient who the surgeon has recently finished working with. Seeing the results first-hand is a good indicator of what you can expect to achieve.
- What training do you have, how long have you been performing this procedure, and how many times have you performed it in the last 12 months? Ask to see photographs of other procedures that the doctor has done.
- What are the risks involved with this procedure? Find out how often they occur and how they will be handled if they do.
- What percentage of patients have had significant complications?
- What is your policy on surgical revisions? Ask about any costs for which you may be responsible if unhappy with the results and require revisions.
- Where will the surgery be performed?

- How long will the procedure take?
- What kind of anaesthesia is used, and what credentials does the person administering it have?
- How will my recovery be monitored immediately after surgery?
- Will I be in pain after surgery and need someone to take me home?
- What is the expected recovery time? Discuss post-operative restrictions on activity, what dressings will be used, and when you can resume work.

Questions to ask before liposuction or body contouring

- Ask to see photos of recent patients whose body type is similar to yours, before and after they had their surgery.
- How will you manage fluid balance during the procedure?
- How much do you expect my skin to contract after the fat is removed?
- What should I expect after the operation in terms of soreness, medication, bathing, and level of activity?

Questions to ask before hair transplants

- Since hair restoration is often done in stages, find out exactly how many sessions you will need, how they will be scheduled and what costs are involved with each.
- What will happen to the result if more hair loss occurs? Will it be necessary to have a second hair transplant in the future if the position of the hairline changes? What clinical studies have been done?

To find a qualified cosmetic surgeon visit www.wlbeauty.com

Other official websites: www.aad.org, www.aafprs.org, www.abplsurg.org, www.asds-net.org, www.aslms.org, www.asoprs.org, www.aao.org/news/eyenet, www.baaps.org.uk, www.plasticsurgery.org, www.surgery.org, www.worldplasticsurgery.org.

index

resources

resources

For more information on beauty secrets, visit Wendy Lewis's website at

www.wlbeauty.com

To learn more about the technologies and therapies discussed in this book, visit:
www.allergan.com, www.botox.com, www.elan.com, www.inamed.com, www.isolagen.com, www.lumenis.com, www.new-fill.com, www.obagi.com, www.orthodermatological.com, www.procyte.com, www.restylane.com, www.sunandskin.com, www.thermage.com and www.wrinklereduction.com.

acknowledgements

The author wishes to thank the following physicians for sharing their expertise for this book:

Fredric Brandt, M.D.; Alastair Carruthers, M.D; Dai Davies, FRCS; Lisa Donofrio, M.D.; Steven Fagien, M.D.; Peter Bela Fodor, M.D.; Bryan Forley, M.D.; Ellen Gendler, M.D.; Roy Geronemus, M.D.; Mitchel Goldman, M.D.; Laurence Kirwan, M.D.; Ted Lockwood, M.D.; Z. Paul Lorenc, M.D.; Nicholas Lowe, M.D.; Alan Matarasso, M.D.; Seth Matarasso, M.D.; Foad Nahai, M.D.; Nicolas Percival, FRCS; Gerald Pitman, M.D.; Rod Rohrich, M.D.; Robin Unger, M.D.; Walter Unger, M.D.; Ken Washenik, M.D.; Patricia Wexler, M.D.; Donald Wood-Smith, M.D.

picture credits

2 *Marie Claire Maison*/Christian Moser; 8 Retna/Michael Putland; 13 Getty Images/James Darell; 18 Getty Images/Chris Craymer; 21 The White Company; 23 Getty Images/Britt Erlanson; 26 Getty Images/Jerome Tisne; 30 Getty Images/Uwe Krejci; 34 Getty Images/Frederic Jorez; 36 Digital Vision; 42 Getty Images/Brian Bailey; 46 Getty Images/David Chambers; 55 Camera Press/*Mise en image*/Nabon; 62 *Marie France*/Alois Beer/Dominique Eveque; 72 Getty Images/Andre Perlstein; 78 Martin Brigdale; 81 Patrick McCleavey; 90 Camera Press/Vital 1562; 98 Photonica/Neo Vision; 103 Gus Filgate; 110 Science Photo Library/Gusto; 121 ImageState; 126 Digital Vision; 132 *Marie Claire Maison*/Pamela Hanson; 144 *Marie Claire Maison*/François Deconinck; 149 Camera Press/*Brigitte*; 158 Getty Images/Peter Nicholson; 161 Getty Images/Chris Bale; 167 Camera Press/*Fair Lady*; 168 IPC Syndication/© *Essentials*/Liz McAulay; 171 Getty Images/David Roth; 177 retna/Jenny Acheson; 180 Getty Images/Bill Ling; 187 Getty Images/Tony Anderson; 192 ImageState/Stock Image; 195 ImageState; 200 Sarah Maingot; 206 Getty Images/Tony Shonnard; 211 retna/Michael Putland; 212 Getty Images/Daniel Bosler; 223 Camera Press/*Fair Lady*; 228 Sarah Maingot; 236 Camera Press/*Brigitte*; 241 Getty Images/David Roth.